A GUIDE TO
LAPAROSCOPIC SURGERY

D1605678

DATE DUE

AUG 1 8 1999		
SEP 0 8 1999		
FEB 2 8 2000		
AUG 1 7 2000		
SEP 0 8 2000		
NOV 2 7 2000		
SEP 13 02		

DEMCO 38-297

A Guide to Laparoscopic Surgery

AZAD NAJMALDIN

MB, ChB, MS, FRCS
Consultant Surgeon
St James's University Hospital
and the General Infirmary
Leeds

PIERRE GUILLOU

BSc, MD, FRCPS (Glasg) Hon, FAMS, FRCS
Professor of Surgery
and Dean of the School of Medicine
University of Leeds
Leeds

b

Blackwell
Science

© 1998 by
Blackwell Science Ltd
Editorial Offices:
Osney Mead, Oxford OX2 oEL
25 John Street, London WC1N 2BL
23 Ainslie Place, Edinburgh EH3 6AJ
350 Main Street, Malden
    MA 02148 5018, USA
54 University Street, Carlton
    Victoria 3053, Australia
10, rue Casimir Delavigne
    75006 Paris, France

Other Editorial Offices:
Blackwell Wissenschafts-Verlag GmbH
Kurfürstendamm 57
10707 Berlin, Germany

Blackwell Science KK
MG Kodenmacho Building
7–10 Kodenmacho Nihombashi
Chuo-ku, Tokyo 104, Japan

First published 1998

Set by Setrite Typesetters, Hong Kong
Printed and bound in Great Britain
by MPG Books Ltd, Bodmin, Cornwall

The Blackwell Science logo is a
trade mark of Blackwell Science Ltd,
registered at the United Kingdom
Trade Marks Registry

For further information on
Blackwell Science, visit our website:
www.blackwell-science.com

DISTRIBUTORS

Marston Book Services Ltd
PO Box 269
Abingdon, Oxon OX14 4YN
(*Orders*: Tel: 01235 465500
        Fax: 01235 465555)

USA
Blackwell Science, Inc.
Commerce Place
350 Main Street
Malden, MA 02148 5018
(*Orders*: Tel: 800 759 6102
             781 388 8250
        Fax: 781 388 8255)

Canada
Login Brothers Book Company
324 Saulteaux Crescent
Winnipeg, Manitoba R3J 3T2
(*Orders*: Tel: 204 837-2987)

Australia
Blackwell Science Pty Ltd
54 University Street
Carlton, Victoria 3053
(*Orders*: Tel: 3 9347 0300
        Fax: 3 9347 5001)

A catalogue record for this title
is available from the British Library

ISBN 0-86542-649-X

Library of Congress
Cataloging-in-publication Data

Najmaldin, Azad.
    A guide to laparoscopic surgery/
    Azad Najmaldin, Pierre Guillou.
        p.   cm.
    ISBN 0-86542-649-X
    1. Laparoscopic surgery—
Technique. 2. Abdomen—
Endoscopic surgery—Technique.
I. Guillou, Pierre J. II. Title.
    [DNLM: 1. Surgical Procedures.
Laparoscopic—methods. 2. Surgical
Procedures, Minimally Invasive—
methods.   WO 505 N162g 1998]
RD540.N29   1998
617'. 05—dc21
DNLM/DLC   98–5987
                                CIP

Contents

Contents

Section 3: Setting up in the operating theatre

Section 4: Laparoscopic procedures

Preface

Wickham noted that three seminal events have indelibly altered surgery: the introduction of anaesthesia, the development of antiseptics, and endoscopy. Laparoscopy is the greatest change in surgical practice this century, and the introduction of laparoscopic cholecystectomy, a decade ago, heralded the development of further laparoscopic techniques in all surgical disciplines. The technique constitutes an important component of any surgeon's work and continues to grow. The importance of understanding proper instrumentation and basic techniques cannot be over emphasized. Having applied the technique of laparoscopy in many aspects of surgery and based on many successful clinical and laboratory courses given nationally and internationally, the authors found that what the trainee needs is a concise, practical, clearly written, easy to follow, and well-illustrated manual. *A Guide to Laparoscopic Surgery* sets out to fulfil these roles. Combining instrumentation, essential basic techniques, common general procedures, and frequently encountered problems and solutions alongside numerous line drawings, this book addresses the needs of surgical trainees in all disciplines, as well as qualified surgeons who have little or no experience with laparoscopy and medical students and theatre staff. While the authors have deliberately forwarded their own strong views as well as other commonly held but differing views, the emphasis throughout is on a clear practical guide to the areas of laparoscopy which the learner will need.

Azad Najmaldin
Pierre Guillou

Section 1
Introduction

Introduction/history

The recent upsurge in the practice of laparoscopic surgery and other forms of 'minimal access surgery' has ushered in a new era of surgical treatment which is having profound effects on surgical management across the various specialities. Although the new approach has been initiated by adult general surgeons and gynaecologists, there is increasing interest in performing laparoscopic/endoscopic procedures in other specialities, such as paediatric surgery, urology, orthopaedic surgery, otorhinolaryngology, cardiovascular surgery, neurosurgery and plastic surgery.

The idea of minimal access surgery is not new; the use of tube and speculum in medicine dates from the earliest days of civilization in Mesopotamia and ancient Greece. Modern endoscopy started in 1805, when Bozzini, an obstetrician from Frankfurt, using candlelight through a tube attempted to examine urethra and vagina in patients. In 1897, Nitze, a urologist from Berlin working with Reinecke, a Berlin optician, and Leiter, a Viennese instrument maker, produced the first usable cystoscope with lenses and platinum wire for illumination. In 1901, von Ott from St. Petersburg reported the first abdominal cavity inspection, by focusing a head mirror into a speculum. A year later Kelling, using a cystoscope after insufflation with filtered air, reported laparoscopy in a living dog to a meeting in Hamburg. In 1910, Jacobaeus, a surgeon from Stockholm, performed laparoscopy and thoracoscopy in a human using a cystoscope. Throughout the 1920s and 1930s, Kalk, the founder of the German School of Laparoscopy, who developed many purpose-designed instruments including oblique-viewing optics, popularized diagnostic laparoscopy in disorders of the liver and biliary tract and opened the way for the development of operative laparoscopy. Subsequently, laparoscopy was developed for gynaecological practice by Palmer (France), Frangenheim and Semm (Germany), Steptoe (UK) and Phillips (USA).

The introduction of fibre-optic light, and the development of the rod lens system by the British physicist Hopkins in 1952, led to dramatic worldwide increase in the use of telescopes in general and laparoscopes in particular.

The origin of modern laparoscopic surgery is derived from the Kiel School in Germany headed by Semm, a gynaecologist. This centre developed and refined many instruments and established most laparoscopic gynaecological procedures currently in practice. Although in use by gynaecologists now for many years, general surgical operations were slow to fall to laparoscopic procedures.

3

Laparoscopically guided gall stone clearance was first performed in an animal model by Frimberger and associates in Germany in 1979. Semm and his group described the technique of a laparoscopic appendicectomy without recourse to mini-laparotomy in 1983. Muehe, a surgeon from Boblingen in Germany introduced cholecystectomy into clinical practice using a modified rectoscope and CO_2 insufflation in 1985. The latest highly significant advance was the introduction of the computer chip video camera in 1986 which ignited the development of today's laparoscopic surgery. In 1987, Mouret, in Lyon (France) was the first surgeon to perform cholecystectomy in the human using standard laparoscopic equipment. The first published report of the current multipuncture cholecystectomy was by Dubois in Paris, France in 1989. Around the same time, the procedure was established by Perissat (Bordeaux, France), Reddick *et al.* (Nashville, USA), Cuschieri and Nathanson (Dundee, UK) and Berci *et al.* (Los Angeles, USA). Since then, the practice of laparoscopic surgical procedures has mushroomed across the various specialities. There can be little doubt that many aspects of the current technology and instrumentation can and will be improved in the near future, thereby increasing the ease of performance and scope of this type of (minimal access) surgery.

Definition

Laparoscopy is the inspection of the peritoneal cavity by means of a telescope introduced through the abdominal wall after creation of a pneumoperitoneum.

Laparoscopic surgery is the execution of established surgical procedures in a way which leads to the reduction of the trauma of access and thereby accelerates the recovery of the patient. Surgical procedures are conducted by remote manipulation and dissection within the closed confines of the abdominal cavity or extraperitoneal space under visual control via telescopes, video cameras and television screens.

Advantages of laparoscopy

In addition to avoiding large, painful access wounds of conventional surgery, laparoscopy allows the operation to be carried out with minimal parietal trauma with the avoidance of exposure, cooling, desiccation, handling, and forced retraction of abdominal tissues and organs. Thus the overall traumatic assault on the patient is reduced drastically, and as a result of this:

- Postoperative pain, ileus and wound complications such as infection and dehiscence are reduced and recovery accelerated.
- Abdominal adhesion formation, which may become the source of recurrent pain, intestinal obstruction and female infertility is reduced.
- Surgically induced immunosuppression, which may have important implications particularly in cancer surgery, is decreased.
- Postoperative chest complications are reduced.
- Cosmetic results are greatly improved.

Other advantages of laparoscopy include:
- Visual enhancement by the magnifying effect of the telescope and improved exposure in places such as the pelvis and subphrenic spaces.
- The greatly reduced contact with patient's blood and body fluid. This has important implications for both patient and surgeon in relation to the transmission of viral diseases.

Disadvantages and limitations of laparoscopy

The main difficulties with laparoscopy emanate from the necessity to insufflate the peritoneal cavity or extraperitoneal space with gas, and access the space via needle and trocar inserted through the abdominal wall. Surgeon-related difficulties include eye and hand co-ordination and the remote nature of the surgical manipulation, loss of direct hand manipulation and tactile feedback and the two-dimensional image provided by the current camera systems. Diathermy injuries are a particular potential hazard. However, appropriate training and experience, open technique laparoscopy, and the development of better instrumentation including three-dimensional video-endoscopy and exploratory ultrasound probe will minimize these difficulties.

The disadvantages of laparoscopy include:
- The need to purchase and maintain expensive high technology equipment.
- Laparoscopic procedures require more technical expertise and take longer, at least initially, than an open approach.
- Potential injury to the vessels and viscera as the result of needle–cannula insertion, inappropriate instrumentation and diathermy burns.
- The insufflation may cause postoperative abdominal pain and shoulder tip pain not uncommonly; and gas embolus, deranged cardiovascular function, tension pneumothorax, and significant hypercarbia very rarely.

- Haemostasis can be difficult to achieve because of technical difficulties and because blood obscures vision by absorbing light.
- Intact organ retrieval, particularly of tumour-containing organs, is seriously limited.

Contraindications/risk factors

Absolute

1 Inability to tolerate general anaesthesia or laparotomy:
   (a) Cardiovascular
   (b) Respiratory
   (c) Uncorrected coagulopathy
   (d) Others.
   Certain laparoscopic procedures, such as diagnostic and minor surgical procedures, may be performed under regional or local anaesthesia.
2 Major haemorrhage requiring life-saving procedures expeditiously:
   (a) Trauma
   (b) Ruptured aneurysm
   (c) Postoperative.
3 Intestinal obstruction (severe distension).

Relative

1 Untrained/inexperienced surgeon.
2 Inadequate equipment/instrument, assistants, time.
3 Severe cardiopulmonary diseases
Risk of CO_2 pneumoperitoneum:
- Increases pressure on diaphragm
- Reduces venous return which leads to lower cardiac output
- Hypercarbia
- Arrythmia
- Head-down position: increases venous pressure in upper half of body.
4 Coagulopathy
Risk of bleeding:
- Bleeding is technically difficult to control laparoscopically because of vessel retraction, the limited ability to apply direct pressure, and limited access.
- The ability to aspirate blood clots is limited by the diameter of the suction probe.

- Blood obscures the view because it absorbs light.
- Direct view is further impaired by brisk haemorrhage splashes on the telescope, and smoke and vapour generated by diathermy.

5 Obesity

Risks: (a) anaesthesia and surgery in general.

(b) Thick abdominal wall:
- Creates difficulty with insertion of needle and trocar.
- Impedes manoeuvrability of the ports/instruments.
- Requires high insufflation pressures.
- Diminishes the visualization of abdominal wall vessels and increases risk of bleeding by direct vessel puncture because of diminished transillumination and excess adipose tissue.

(c) Thick omentum and mesentery further impedes manipulation and visibility.

6 Abdominal wall pathology. Hernia: risks:

(a) hernia creates difficulty with insertion of needle and trocar in conventional port sites such as the umbilicus with the consequent risk of injury to the bowel.

(b) Obstructed hernia:
- there is difficulty with laparoscopic reduction;
- pneumoperitoneum further compromises the circulation of the strangulated organ.

(c) Embryonic remnants such as the vitello-intestinal duct and urachus may cause difficulty during placement of needles and ports.

7 Intra-abdominal pathology. Abdominal adhesions: risks:
- injury to bowel, omentum, mesentery and vessels at needle/cannula insertion;
- difficulty in creating an effective pneumoperitoneum;
- poor view from excessive scarring;
- prolongs the procedure because of the need for adhesiolysis.

Intestinal obstructions (mild/moderate distension)

Risks: distended loops:
- injury to bowel and mesentery at needle/trocar insertion;
- diminishes view and working space;
- impedes manoeuvrability of and around the intestine.

Advanced peritonitis: risks:
- intestinal obstruction/ileus (as above);
- poor view and inability to localize the site of perforation by fibrinous adhesions.

Significant aneurysm

Risk: bleeding from needle/trocar introduction.

Large benign liver, spleen and other abdominal mass: risks:
- injury for needle/trocar introduction and instrument manoeuvre;
- diminishes view and working space.

Pregnancy: risks:
  (a) Mother and fetus.
  - general anaesthetic and operative;
  - unknown effect of pneumoperitoneum and CO_2.
  (b) Pregnant uterus:
  - injury from needle/trocar placement and instrument manipulation;
  - diminishes view and working space.

Malignant diseases: risks:
  (a) inadequate access.
  (b) Restricted intact organ retrieval;
  - contamination may preclude histological staging.
  (c) Gas insufflation may cause spread of malignant cells.

Combined laparoscopy and open surgery

This approach combines the inherent minimally invasive nature of laparoscopy, and the speed and simplicity of open surgery in situations where the laparoscopic approach alone may prove technically difficult and time consuming. Current indications include:
- Inexperienced surgeon.
- Laparoscopy as a preliminary measure to diagnose and localize the pathology:
  (a) Trauma
  (b) Acute and chronic abdominal pain
  (c) Peritonitis
  (d) Malignancy
  (e) Intussusception
  (f) Jaundice
  (g) Undescended testes and intersex anomalies
  (h) Others.
- Combined procedures:
  (a) Abdominoperineal approaches for anorectal surgery and colon pullthrough.
  (b) Abdominothoracocervical approaches for gastro-oesophageal surgery.
  (c) Laparoscopic-assisted vaginal hysterectomy
  (d) Upper and lower urinary tract surgery when nephrectomy is

required with a form of bladder reconstruction or reimplantation of ureter.
  (e) Abdominoscrotal approaches to the testes.
• Intact organ retrieval:
  (a) Cancer treatment
  (b) Large organs (spleen, kidney)
  (c) Large segment bowel resection such as total colectomy.
• Manipulation, resection and anastomosis especially in intestinal surgery and rectopexy.
• Complications of laparoscopic surgery.

Physiological changes during laparoscopy

Although the surgical technique of laparoscopic surgery is of a minimally invasive nature, a number of physiological changes occur as a result of creating a CO_2 pneumoperitoneum/pneumoextraperitoneum, and postural changes involved in patient positioning. These changes may be particularly noticeable in elderly and very young patients, and significant in those with pre-existing diseases such as cardiovascular, pulmonary and neurological disorders. In addition, other pathophysiological changes related to access and instrument injuries leading to bleeding, gas embolism or peritonitis may occur. It must be remembered that conventional open surgery too, has significant effects on body physiology as the result of wound related trauma and pain, pulmonary dysfunction, bowel dysfunction from exposure and handling, endocrine and metabolic changes, as well as postural changes required for optimal surgical access.

Respiratory changes

• Changes in pulmonary function occur with the administration of any general anaesthetic.
• Functional residual capacity (FRC) is reduced by diaphragmatic displacement and splinting, and changes in intrathoracic blood volume develop as the result of pneumoperitoneum and Trendelenburg positioning. This results in small airway collapse which in turn leads to atelectasis, pulmonary shunting and hypoxaemia.
• Diaphragmatic displacement will also lead to a significant rise in peak airway pressure, increase in physiological dead space and a reduction of up to 50% in total lung compliance. Despite these, only minor modifications in gas exchange occurs unless there is pre-existing cardiopulmonary disease when greater changes can occur.

- During insufflation, CO_2 is readily absorbed into the blood stream, where most then diffuses into the red cells, where hydration to carbonic acid and subsequent ionization occur, helped by the buffering capacity of Hb for hydrogen ion. HCO_3^- ion is then released into the plasma in exchange for Cl^- ion. during CO_2 insufflation therefore, end-tidal CO_2 (Et CO_2) and arterial ($Paco_2$) would rise rapidly by around 8–10 mmHg and then plateau at a new equilibrium after around 35 min. Unless this excess CO_2 can be removed by adequate ventilation, significant hypercarbia and respiratory acidosis will occur. This may cause tachycardia, dysrhythmias, and an increase in myocardial oxygen consumption. In healthy individuals, normocarbia may be achieved by a 25% increase in minute ventilation through an intubated trachea.

- Current evidence suggests that in healthy individuals pulmonary function is better preserved after laparoscopic surgery and changes that take place may be of shorter duration compared with open surgery. Forced vital capacity (FVC) and forced expiratory volume in 1 second (FEV_1) at 24 h are reduced by 25% after laparoscopic cholecystectomy compared with a 48% reduction after open surgery. Changes in FRC and arterial Po_2 at 24 h are small and significant clinically while arterial Pco_2 is unchanged. However, these changes may be more significant in patients with underlying pulmonary dysfunction.

- Respiratory failure may occur if patients are allowed to breath spontaneously. Hypoventilation may occur as a result of drug-related respiratory depression, and diaphragmatic displacement and splinting.

- Excessive airway pressure may result in pulmonary barotrauma which may compromise cardiac output, especially if bronchospasm occurs, in the very obese, and in steep Trendelenburg positions. Therefore attempts should be made to maintain airway pressure below 40 cmH$_2$O by manipulating tidal volume, and respiratory pattern and frequency.

- Pneumothorax may occur from gas tracking along the tissue planes or surgically traumatized pleura, undetected diaphragmatic hernia, pulmonary barotrauma or rupture of an emphysematous bulla. An unexpected increase in end tidal CO_2, increase in airway pressure, reduction in pulmonary compliance, falling oxygen saturation and reduced airway entry on auscultation, should alert the anaesthetist to the possibility of pneumothorax. Despite the potential problems, tension pneumoperitoneum is usually well tolerated requiring only moderate increase in oxygen concentration and minute ventilation in the majority of patients. However, any major problems with oxygenation must be treated aggressively with deflation of the abdomen, chest X-ray, and thoracocentesis, if appropriate.

• Bronchial intubation may result from upward displacement of the trachea during high pressure peritoneal insufflation. This may lead to bronchospasm, hypoxia and atelectasis. The position of the endotracheal tube should always be checked intra-operatively.

• Aspiration of gastric contents may occur from increased intra-abdominal pressure, change in posture and manipulation of the stomach. The risk can be reduced by appropriate nasogastric and endotracheal tube placement.

• Clinical gas embolus, a potentially lethal complication, is exceedingly rare. It is usually caused by accidental intravascular injection of insufflation gas through a misplaced Veress needle, forcing of gas into a vein splinted open, or air from a cooled laser tip. The physiological effects will depend on the rate and volume of gas introduced and tend to be less dramatic with CO_2 than with air, as the former is more soluble in blood. Gas embolization may be a delayed phenomenon as the result of trapping in the portal circulation. Using transoesophageal echo sonography, subclinical CO_2 embolization appears commonly without significant effects on the cardiovascular system. While a slow infusion of CO_2 is readily absorbed across the capillary–alveolar membrane, higher rates may cause obstruction of pulmonary arterioles which provokes plugging, activation of the clotting cascade and release of chemical mediators resulting in bronchospasm and pulmonary oedema. Large infusion rates of 3 ml/kg or more, may cause an airlock at the right atrium and ventricle leading to cardiovascular collapse. Cerebral gas embolism may occur as a result of gas entering the systemic circulation via a patent cardiac foramen or through the pulmonary capillary system and can result in neurological dysfunction.

The outcome of massive gas embolism depends on early detection and treatment. Transoesophageal echo-monitoring, 'mill wheel' murmur on auscultation and decreased end-tidal CO_2 are sensitive diagnostic measures. Treatment should include discontinuation of gas flow and desufflation, head down tilt to minimize the outflow obstruction of the right side of the heart, attempts to aspirate gas from the right side of heart if a central venous line is available, and intravenous fluid to prevent hypotension.

Cardiovascular changes

• Changes caused by anaesthesia and respiratory alterations.
• Peritoneal insufflation with or without Trendelenburg position may result in:

(a) An increase in mean arterial pressure through a significantly increased systemic vascular resistance.

(b) A fall in cardiac output caused by direct pressure on the inferior vena cava and pelvic veins which reduces venous return. However, this effect may be partly compensated for by blood pushed out of the inferior vena cava and splanchnic bed into the central venous space.

(c) An increase in systemic vascular resistance by mechanical compression of the aorta and splanchnic vessels, and the release of humoral factors such as catecholamines, prostaglandins, renin-angiotensin and vasopressin.

(d) Increased cardiac filling pressures, central venous pressure and pulmonary capillary wedge pressure caused by the central redistribution of blood or the increased intrathoracic pressure.

The effects of pneumoperitoneum are more marked during the initial 30 min of insufflation.

- Reverse Trendelenburg position reduces venous return and cardiac filling pressure through gravitational effects, which in turn reduce cardiac index and mean arterial pressure. The combined effects of anaesthesia, reverse Trendelenburg and pneumoperitoneum of 15 mmHg CO_2 produce a reduction in cardiac output of a much as 30%.
- Left ventricular function would appear well preserved despite changes in loading conditions and posture.

Renal changes

The increase in renal vascular resistance, decreased cardiac output and rise in vasopressin levels may all lead to a reduction in renal blood flow and glomerular filtration rate.

Electrolyte balance

Prolonged CO_2 pneumoperitoneum produces a trend for serum potassium to increase but not to a clinically significant level under normal conditions.

Metabolic changes

The metabolic response to surgery is complex and mediated by neuroendocrine stimulation and inflammatory mediators, which in turn are activated by tissue trauma. It appears that, overall, the neuroendocrine response to laparoscopy is similar to that of open surgery, but the extent of the surgical trauma is less in the laparoscopy patients. The former may be caused by afferent neuronal stimulation from the pneumoperitoneum.

Anaesthesia during laparoscopy

General anaesthesia with intubation and controlled ventilation, is generally the preferred anaesthetic technique for the vast majority of laparoscopic procedures. Laparoscopy under epidural analgesia or local anaesthetic techniques, is unpopular because of patient discomfort associated with pneumoperitoneum and postural changes, the need to avoid respiratory embarrassment, hypercarbia, and aspiration, and the possible risks of bleeding, gas embolus and arrythmia.

- The patient's age, size, pre-existing illnesses and contraindications to laparoscopy, should all be carefully assessed.
- The anaesthetist must be prepared to encounter complications such as major bleeding, gas embolus, and pneumothorax.
- Adequate monitoring will allow the early detection of complications.
- Nasogastric aspiration via a tube improves access in the upper abdomen and minimizes the risk of pulmonary aspiration.
- A bladder catheter improves access in the lower abdomen and allows monitoring of urinary output.
- Ensure adequate venous access and consideration should be given to the necessity for a central venous catheter and arterial line.
- Complete muscle relaxation is necessary to avoid any sudden movement by the patient which may be hazardous.
- Nitrous oxide may cause practical problems related to intestinal distension and has the theoretical disadvantages of increasing the size of a gas embolus and the chance of combustion by diffusion into the abdominal cavity.
- Maintain patient core temperature, particularly during laparoscopy in the elderly and children, and the more prolonged procedures.

Postoperative management

In uncomplicated laparoscopic procedures pain and nausea are the two major causes of postoperative morbidity in the first 12–24 h. Pain after laparoscopic surgery is less severe and of shorter duration than after open surgery. The sites of pain are:
- wound

- shoulder tip
- generalized abdominal.

The latter two are thought to be caused either by mechanical stretching from the pneumoperitoneum or direct irritation from CO_2. The frequency and severity of pain from these sources may be reduced by using a low initial flow rate and pressure of CO_2 insufflation, and complete aspiration of the pneumoperitoneum at the end of the procedure.

Wound pain may be managed initially with local infiltration of local anaesthetic agents. Non-steroidal anti-inflammatory drugs may be useful in controlling pain. The choice of anaesthetic technique and agents can significantly influence the development of post-operative nausea and vomiting.

Section 2
Equipment, instruments, basic techniques, problems and solutions

Equipment

Camera

High quality visualization of the operative field is essential during laparoscopic surgery. The modern silicon chip lightweight camera has a zoom lens, automatic colour setting, high speed shutter to eliminate over-exposure, and is easily sterilized both by ethylene oxide gas and gluteraldelyde. Some models have buttons mounted on the camera piece itself for adjusting the sensitivity to light, and to activate the video recorder and printer.

The number of pixels on a chip determines the resolution capacity. A single chip camera (450 lines per inch) provides good quality imaging, while a three chip camera (700 lines per inch) provides better resolution and colour accuracy but is more expensive, heavier and bulkier to hand grip. Both cameras produce two-dimensional imaging. However, prototype three-dimensional cameras which have the potential to make laparoscopy easier, quicker, less prone to error and more applicable to advanced procedures are now under development.

An ideal camera has the following characteristics:
- High quality resolution and colour accuracy.
- Has an automatic high speed iris shutter to prevent over-exposure, a zoom capability, and does not require focusing.
- Moisture proof, light in weight and easy hand grip.
- Compatible with available telescopes, durable and inexpensive.

Monitor

Although endoscopic surgery can be performed with only one monitor, two sets are preferable so that the surgeon and assistant on either side of the operating table can see along a direct line. A standard monitor with resolution of 450 lines/inch matches the picture of a one chip camera, whereas a high resolution monitor with 700 lines/inch suits the character of a three chip camera. Once a monitor has been set, it should not be touched.

Light source

Most of the light sources currently available are capable of manual and automatic adjustment for optimum light required for each procedure. The quality of the light is extremely important for the accurate transmission of colour and imaging. The illumination required in laparoscopy is best provided by powerful light sources, such as xenon. Losses of a significant percentage of the transmitted light energy are expected along the flexible fibre optic cable, telescope, and each interface from source to body cavity; low powered sources are usually inadequate. The light maintains its sensitivity with a minimum of heat conduction to the telescope, hence the term 'cold light' is used. However, the heat produced at the end of the fibre optic or telescope can be sufficient to burn the drape, patient or internal organs if there is prolonged contact.

Documentation device

A video recorder with or without still image photography is important for documentation, learning and teaching.

Imaging trolley

A purpose designed trolley not only accommodates the monitor at a convenient height, but also the camera control unit, light source, video recorder, printer, suction irrigation device, insufflator and ultrasound screen. Such a trolley reduces the number of trailing wires and cables on the floor and allows easy manoeuvrability around the theatre and operating table.

Telescope

The laparoscopic telescope has two channels (Fig. 1), one channel being the optical 'viewing channel', and the second is the glass fibres that transmit light. The optical channel, comprises of rod-lenses, the 'Hopkins rod lens system'. In this system, light is transmitted through glass columns and refracted through intervening air spaces. The endoscope does not simply magnify the image as does a

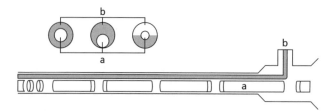

Fig. 1 Longitudinal and transverse section of telescope. (a) Rod-lenses with short intervening air spaces; (b) Light glass fibre.

microscope. However, objects are magnified at a certain distance from the end of the telescope.

The glass fibre has a centre of glass, and an outer glass sleeve with a lower light diffraction index. This property allows near total light transmission to the end of the glass fibre (Fig. 2).

A variety of designs and types of laparoscopic telescope are available for use. Diameters range from 2.5 to 12 mm. A 10 mm scope transmits nearly four and 10 times more light compared with a 5 mm and a 3 mm telescope, respectively, and it therefore provides a better view.

The spectrum of viewing angles ranges from 0° forward viewing to 70° oblique (Fig. 3). The most commonly used telescope is a zero degree telescope. However, the telescope with an angled lens (30° or 45°) can offer more versatility by allowing a combination of forward and lateral viewing.

An operating telescope (Fig. 4), incorporates both a telescope

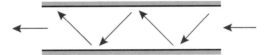

Fig. 2 Light transmission through glass fibre.

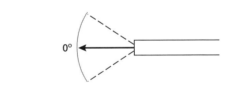

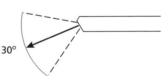

Fig. 3 Telescopes 0° and 30° viewing angles.

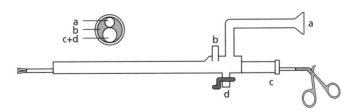

Fig. 4 Operating telescope. Cross-section and lateral view: (a) optic channel; (b) light channel; (c) instrument channel with an instrument *in situ*; (d) gas port.

and a working channel in a 10mm instrument. The disadvantages of this type of instrument are a restricted view (comparable to that of a 5 mm telescope) and the difficulty in manipulating the instrument in the same line of view.

Problems and solutions with imaging and viewing

High quality imaging of the operative field is mandatory for laparoscopic procedures. To avoid problems with imaging and its consequences:

• Use high quality and matching equipment, connections and instruments.

• Become familiar with the ways equipment is set, connected, used and maintained.

• Take advantage of accessory equipment, connections and instruments which are available for difficult circumstances.

• Ensure the availability of properly trained assistants, back-up equipment and engineers.

Problems with imaging are not an uncommon occurrence and can happen at the beginning or at any other stages during the procedure. They can be frustrating, time consuming and dangerous.

1   Total blackout of one or more screens:
   (a) Faulty equipment in a particular light source and cables;
   (b) Improper, loose or unmatched connections.

2   Unexpected differential in quality of imaging in between two screens:
   (a) Loose or unmatched connection;
   (b) Reset monitor.

3   Interference on screen: this may be caused by a diathermy unit.
   (a) Position and plug diathermy unit furthest away from monitor and cameral control unit.
   (b) Keep camera cable separate from diathermy cable.

4   Glare: this happens as the result of disturbed balance of light intensity detected by the camera.
   (a) High light output;
   (b) Malfunctioning automatic/manual iris shutter of camera;
   (c) Shiny metal instruments reflecting light.

5   Dark images:
   (a) Low light output from light source, small inadequate light cable, or small telescope.
   (b) The automatic light sensor of the camera reacts to the high reflection of light from shiny metal instruments by darkening the view of the monitor.

(c) Blood in the peritoneal cavity absorbs light and reduces the amount of reflected light. Regular suction and irrigation of blood will maximize illumination.

6 Blurred or poor quality colour and image:

(a) Camera focusing inadequate.

(b) An accurate spectrum of colours requires automatic or manual white balancing, prior to inserting the telescope.

(c) Variables such as the length, diameter and quality of the flexible fibre optic can affect the quality of the imaging.

(d) Damaged telescope.

(e) Loose connections, debris and moisture at all interfaces distort the image. The interfaces between camera lead and camera control unit, parts of the camera, camera and telescope, tip of telescope, light cable and light source, light cable and telescope must be kept clean and dry.

(f) Contaminated tip of the telescope with peritoneal fluid such as blood, pus, irrigated fluid. A quick wipe or rinse inside the peritoneal cavity or outside the cannula should solve this problem.

7 Fogging: condensation only occurs when warmer moist air is allowed to condense on colder surfaces. Components which are of different materials can heat up and cool down at different rates. Condensation may take place within the camera, the camera to telescope couple and at the end of the telescope.

(a) A non-moisture-proof camera must be kept dry.

(b) The light cable, telescope and camera (if sterilized) should be kept warm by rinsing in warm water. Telescopes may be placed in specialized warmers.

(c) The use of camera drapes maintains the camera at room temperature, helping to minimize temperature differences.

(d) Dry all interfaces prior to use (camera to telescope, light to telescope, end of telescope).

(e) Anti-fogging fluids are helpful but expensive.

(f) Transfer the CO_2 gas lead to a cannula other than the one carrying the telescope, because the cold gas tends to enhance condensation.

8 Smoke and debris (snow storm): occur as a result of excess diathermy use, especially with monopolar current. Regular desufflation of the peritoneal cavity via cannula valves clears the space.

9 Inexperienced camera operator: the camera must be focused on the operative field in a steady hand, and should move only when it is necessary.

10 Problems with access: inappropriately positioned cannula carrying the telescope.

(a) Telescope too far from the target operative field. Use an alternative site for telescope.

(b) View obstructed by bowel or other organs. An angled telescope (30–70°) often improves imaging.

11 Theatre set-up and monitor position:

(a) The surgeon, assistants and camera operator on either side of the operating table should see along a direct line with monitors at a comfortable eye level.

(b) The reflection of the theatre light (or even outside light) from the surface of the video monitors may disturb viewing.

Sterilization and maintenance of optics and camera

Equipment and instruments that come into contact with patients, directly or indirectly, must be sterile. The steam autoclave, which is one of the most reliable methods of sterilization causes stress and corrosion on the equipment. Therefore, the laparoscopic surgery camera, light cable and the telescopes are usually sterilized in a suitable solution. Gluteraldehyde, a widely used sterilizing solution, may also cause corrosion particularly of the camera and its lead, and represents an occupational hazard for the staff. The use of camera drapes alleviates the need for sterilization and undoubtedly prolongs the life of the camera. Nowadays, some manufacturers have introduced autoclavable telescopes.

The optics and camera are expensive to repair and replace; therefore great care must be taken with their handling.

• Camera lead and light cables are easily broken and should not be bent or caught under the wheels of trolleys.

• Use camera drapes whenever possible.

• Telescopes are easily chipped and bent. Gently introduce telescopes through metal cannulae, and support small diameter telescopes at both camera and cannula levels.

Instruments and access

Perhaps the most important step in any successful laparoscopic procedure is access. To achieve access one needs:

• A sound knowledge of anatomy;
• An understanding of the equipment and instruments necessary;
• A safely created pneumoperitoneum;
• Appropriate size, site and safely placed primary and secondary cannulae;
• Adequate use of retraction.

There is no doubt that the most difficult and dangerous steps in laparoscopic surgery are the insertion of the Veress needle and the first large cannula (closed method laparoscopy). For this reason, it is important to be able to perform open insertions of the primary cannula using the Fielding or Hasson techniques, and many surgeons have now abandoned the Veress needle.

Anatomy

The fundamental principle of endo-anatomy is that structures and their relations are not in any way different anatomically. The important difference is that laparoscopy affords the surgeon an unfamiliar view or orientation of anatomical structures. Thus, a thorough appreciation of structural relations in three dimensions is essential for the accurate and safe dissection of tissues.

Nearly all laparoscopic cameras currently used give a two-dimensional image of a three-dimensional anatomical object. It is, therefore, important to identify ways in which three-dimensional anatomical relationships of structures can be appreciated on the screen. Tissue folds and protrusions often give rise to shadows and contours. These subtle differences may be used to gauge distance of tissues and their proximity to one another. Colour appreciation may also help in the identification of anatomical structures. Once positively identified, the surgeon can then further dissect and identify adjacent structures using a sound knowledge of anatomical relationships.

Despite the development of laparoscopic surgery from open surgical techniques, the steps undertaken to complete a particular procedure sometimes can be radically different when using the laparoscope, as in inguinal hernia repair. Here, the need for sound anatomical knowledge is essential. To further complicate matters, adhesion, inflammation, enlarged, distorted or displaced organ or minor bleeding in the operative field can all act to hinder the laparoscopic access and view of anatomical structures.

Meticulous technique, adherence to defined tissue planes, avoidance of bleeding, and scrupulous haemostasis are important in maintaining awareness and confidence of anatomical position during laparoscopic surgery.

Insufflator

A high flow automatic electronic insufflator should have four clearly visible and easily adjustable gauges; one indicates the rate of flow of CO_2 into the abdomen (up to 10 l/min), one monitors CO_2 cylinder pressure, one records the total volume of gas delivered and above all a fourth must constantly monitor the intra-abdominal pressure and stop the flow of gas automatically once the preselected abdominal pressure is reached. It is also important that the device has a clearly audible alarm to signal all malfunctions especially that of excess intra-abdominal pressure.

• Before starting any procedure, check that the machine is in a working condition, and the attached CO_2 cylinder contains sufficient gas for the completion of the procedure.

• Place a gas filter in between the insufflator and the sterile tubing.

• Ensure that the pressure limit does not exceed 10–14 mmHg.

Veress needle

The Veress needle is a long needle with a blunt hollow spring loaded trocar in its centre. The blunt trocar springs back at and through the resistance of the abdominal wall, and springs out again to protect the viscera from the needle once the resistance disappears within the abdominal cavity (Fig. 5). Gas flows through the hollow trocar to create the initial pneumoperitoneum.

• The Veress needle may be of the reusable type: with use, cleaning and sterilization, this needle can become blunt and its spring mechanism inefficient. However, it is cost-effective.

• The disposable Veress needle is a single use needle which should have a sharp tip and an effective spring.

• Before use the patency of the needle should be checked by a flushing with a syringe, and the spring mechanism tested by pushing against resistance, but care must be taken not to damage the sharp tip.

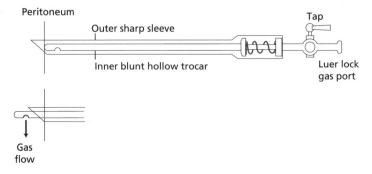

Fig. 5 The Veress needle and its mechanism of action.

Cannulae and trocars

The cannula or 'port' is a tubular device through which operative access is obtained. All cannulae, have a sharp trocar (except the Hasson cannula which is blunt) to facilitate passage through the abdominal wall, and a valve or membrane to prevent gas leaking when no instrument is in place (Fig. 6). Most cannulae also have a rubber seal at the top through which telescopes and instruments may be passed without the loss of pneumoperitoneum. Some sharp pointed trocars have a central channel which allows an audible release of gas when the tip of the trocar penetrates the parietal peritoneum indicating that the trocar is appropriately placed. Not all cannulae have a side port for insufflation. Cannulae are available from 3 to 20 mm in diameter (5 mm and 10 mm are the most commonly used). The tip of the cannula can be straight or bevelled. The latter may be advanced through the abdominal wall with greater ease, but reduces the functioning distance available between the cannula and the operative field which may be important when the cannula is placed close to the operative field, or in paediatric surgery (Fig. 7).

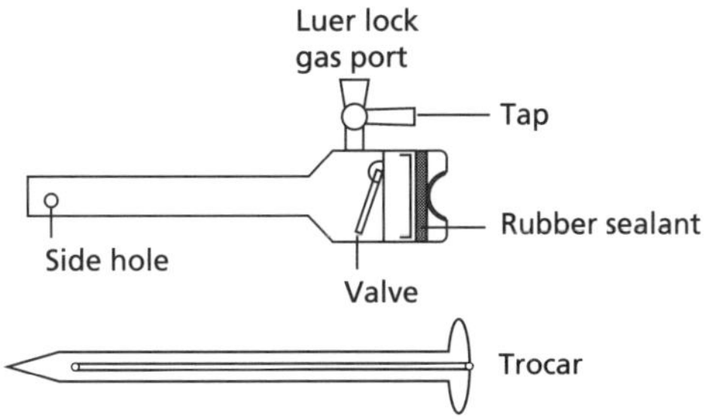

Fig. 6 Cannula and trocar (trocar with a central channel).

Fig. 7 Cannula tip with a grasper *in situ*. Note how the reduced functioning distance in the bevelled cannula prevents the grasping forceps from being fully opened.

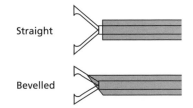

The types of valves used for cannulae are (Fig. 8):

1 Flap valve:

• The majority of cannulae, disposable and reusable, have this type of valve system with an outside valve lever to ensure that it can be easily opened.

• They lose their gas seal with use or in the presence of trapped tissue particles.

• Without a suture introducer (Fig. 9), needles and sutures may get caught in the flap valve. This problem is minimized by keeping the valve fully opened during insertion and removal of suturing materials.

• Some metal flap valves on reusable cannulae may cause damage to the tip of telescope and the insulation sheath of instruments unless the valve is kept fully opened during the introduction and withdrawal.

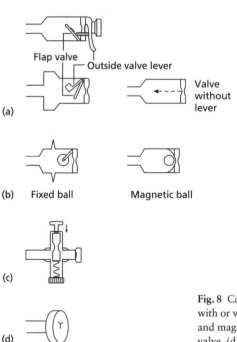

Fig. 8 Cannula valve. (a) Flap valves with or without external lever. (b) Fixed and magnetic ball valves. (c) Trumpet valve. (d) Membrane valve.

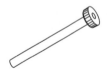

Fig. 9 Suture introducer.

- During withdrawal of instruments, especially curved tip instruments, sutures, slings and pledget swabs, a flap valve may cause accidental removal of the cannulae unless the valve is kept fully opened and the cannula is fixed by hand, a self-retaining collar device, or a suture.
2 Ball valve 'fixed or magnet':
  - Not a popular system, though easy to use.
  - Requires a suture introducing device when the cannula is used for suturing. This is because it has no outside valve lever.
3 Trumpet valve (metal reusable only):
  - Seals very well, but to move instruments and telescopes within the cannulae, the valve needs to be depressed.
  - Not good for suturing without a suture introducer.
  - Can damage telescopes and instruments relatively easily; therefore, it is not a popular system.
4 Soft plastic membrane 'diaphragm': this consists of a thick, usually silastic, membrane with a Y shape cut in its centre which acts as a valve and sealant. This membrane can, sometimes, accept different sizes of instruments without reducers.

Three styles of trocars are available: blunt, conical and pyramidal (Fig. 10).
1 Blunt: these are used during the open technique of cannula insertion or replacement of a removed/dislodged cannula.
2 Conical:
  - Less traumatic to tissue;
  - Less gaping of the wound in the abdominal wall after removal;
  - Requires greater force for tissue penetration and consequently increases the risk of visceral injury.
3 Pyramidal: this has a more effective cutting point, therefore less force is required for tissue penetration, and consequently reduces the risk of visceral injury, but increases the chance of abdominal wall vessel injury.

A variety of disposable and reusable cannulae are available with a spring loaded sheath which automatically covers the sharp trocar point and locks in place when the abdominal wall is penetrated.

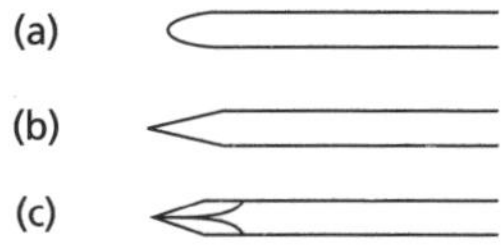

(a)

(b)

(c)

Fig. 10 Trocars. (a) Blunt; (b) conical; (c) pyramidal.

When used properly, this system undoubtedly reduces, but does not abolish, the risk of injury to intra-abdominal structures (Fig. 11a). The safety shield mechanism is influenced by: the length of the sharp cutting tip of the trocar which has to pass the peritoneal layer before the shield descends, the thickness of the rim of the sheath, and the size of the incision made for introduction of the cannula/trocar. The shield may snag at any level of the abdominal wall (skin, muscle, fascia, peritoneum) and remains unable to snap forward after the sharp tip has already entered the peritoneal cavity (Fig. 11b).

Other safety trocar mechanisms are also available, but have not yet become popular.

Cannulae/trocars are available in two main forms:

1   Reusable cannulae/trocar:
   • May be metal (conductive for electrical charges) or plastic/ceramic (non-conductive);
   • The plastic/ceramic type possesses a safety shield;
   • Have a long working life and are therefore cost-effective;
   • Require meticulous sterilization after each use;
   • Require care and maintenance of the valve system and safety shield mechanism;
   • The sharp tip of the trocar may require resharpening or changing now and then;
   • The top rubber sealant needs to be changed regularly, because it can be cut by the trocar or instruments causing a gas leak;
   • To reduce the effective internal diameter of the cannula, reducing sleeves and diaphragms are available (Fig. 12).
2   Disposable cannulae/trocar:
   • May be plastic or metal;

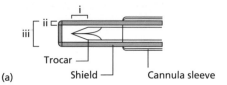

(a)

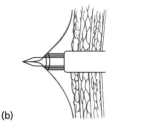

(b)

Fig. 11 (a) Safety shield. The mechanism is influenced by: (i) length of the sharp tip of the trocar; (ii) the thickness of the rim of the shield; (iii) incision which should match the outer diameter of the shield. (b) The shield is caught at the peritoneum.

- Are always pristine, perfectly sterilized, and problems with mechanical malfunction are very rare;
- Most have a safety shield mechanism;
- Are expensive and the high cost for a single use is the only disadvantage;
- Reducing diaphragms are available to reduce the internal working diameter of the cannula (some have built in reducer).

Anchoring device

Anchoring stitches or devices may prevent cannula dislodgement (Fig. 13). These are particularly helpful in thin or paediatric patients, and in protracted laparoscopic procedures. Anchoring stitches are easy and effective, but do not prevent cannulae falling into the abdominal cavity which can be frustrating during dissection and suturing. Likewise, inflatable balloon and wing Malécot arrangements, which

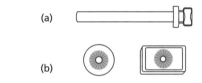

Fig. 12 Reducing devices. (a) Sleeve for reusable cannula; (b) diaphragm for reusable and disposable cannulae.

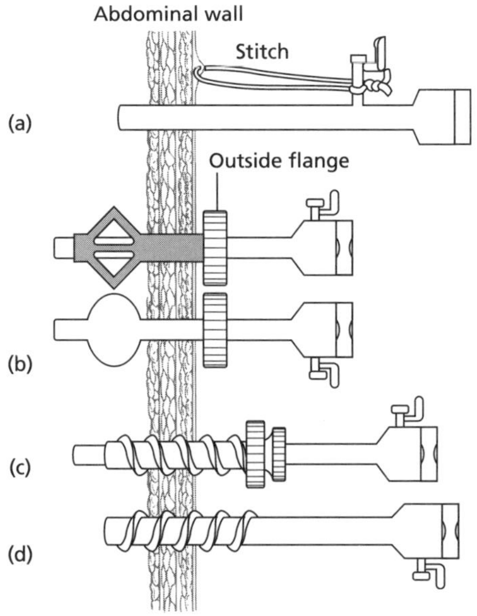

Fig. 13 Anchoring device. (a) Stitch through the skin tied to gas port; (b) Malécot or balloon arrangement (disposable cannulae only); (c) anchoring by threads (spiral retaining collar) with a cannula *in situ*; (d) anchoring feature built onto cannula.

are available on some disposable cannulae, prevent cannulae falling out but not falling in (without an outside flange).

A specially designed reusable or disposable sheath with anchoring threads (spiral retaining collar) may hold the cannula in place. However, they do not completely abolish cannula displacement and they traumatize the wound edges and allow gaping of the hole in the abdominal wall after cannula removal, thereby increasing the risks of infection and herniation through the wound. Some disposable cannulae have an anchoring feature built into the cannula.

Creation of pneumoperitoneum/access

All laparoscopic surgery requires that the peritoneal cavity be turned into a space to enable diagnostic or therapeutic procedures to be performed. This space is created by either mechanical retraction of the abdominal wall (gasless laparoscopy) or distension with gas insufflation (pneumoperitoneum). The gases that can be used for insufflation are CO_2, O_2, air, nitrous oxide, helium or argon.

Oxygen and air support combustion and have a higher risk of gas embolism. Nitrous oxide has unpredictable rapid absorption, risk of gas embolism and hazards to the health of the theatre staff from leaked gas. CO_2 is the most commonly used gas for pneumoperitoneum. It is safe and rapidly cleared by the lungs. CO_2 has no optical distortion, suppresses combustion, is readily available and inexpensive.

Although the vast majority of laparoscopic procedures have been carried out using a pneumoperitoneum created with CO_2, the technique is not without problems. Creation and maintenance of pressurized gas within the abdominal cavity have definite physiological effects on the cardiovascular and pulmonary systems, and exposes the patient to the risk, albeit very small, of gas embolism (see Physiological changes (page 9) and Complications (page 38)). Positive pressure CO_2 insufflation has also been linked to tumour seeding mechanisms.

A pneumoperitoneum may be created by two methods: the closed method using a Veress needle and/or primary cannula; or open method using Hasson's technique or its modifications (Fielding). Whatever method is chosen and before starting the operation, make sure that:

• The insufflator is properly functioning and set at the desired level of gas flow and pressure; and the gas cylinder contains sufficient gas.

- There is a sufficiently long gas lead 'tube' (connected gas filter is recommended).
- Sufficient number and different sizes of cannulae/trocars and reducers are available.
- If reusable items used: Veress needle (close method laparoscopy only), and cannulae and trocars are sharp and functioning properly.
- If disposable items used, their functions are tested.
- The patient is appropriately positioned (usually supine) and prepared.
- The abdomen is inspected and palpated for the size and thickness of the abdomen; previous scars; enlarged organs such as liver and spleen; abnormal masses such as tumours, aneurysms, inflammation, and hernias and bladder.
- A palpable bladder should be drained. An indwelling catheter is only necessary to monitor urine output and for better access during pelvic surgery. Routine catheterization is unnecessary for most basic laparoscopic procedures but may be required for some advanced procedures.
- A nasogastric tube is placed in all cases of upper abdominal procedures. This helps towards safer and better access, and minimizes the risk of aspiration.
- A patient with a scarred abdomen should undergo a pre-operative ultrasound examination. An experienced examiner can indicate the site of abdominal scar, allowing a safe insertion of the cannula.
- Whenever the need arises, the plan/procedure should be converted to open surgery and the patient is consented for this eventuality.

Gasless laparoscopy

To avoid the disadvantages of CO_2 insufflation, devices are available for lifting the anterior abdominal wall to facilitate gasless laparoscopy. Some devices provide tenting of the anterior abdominal wall by traction of the skin and subcutaneous tissues (U shaped retractor or subcutaneous wires), whereas others lift up the entire abdominal wall via an intraperitoneal retractor (wires, or L, T, or fan shaped retractor) (Fig. 14). Despite these inventions the technique of gasless laparoscopy has not yet achieved wide popularity.

Potential advantages are:
- Avoids physiological alterations associated with CO_2 pneumoperitoneum;
- Minimizes the risk of gas embolization;
- Avoids the need and maintenance of a gas-tight operating environment;

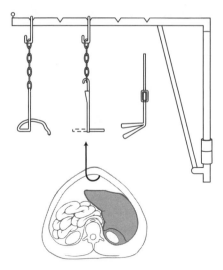

Fig. 14 Devices for lifting anterior abdominal wall.

- May allow the use of conventional instruments;
- Is a safe alternative method of laparoscopy in high risk patients. Disadvantages are:
- The overall exposure is usually inferior to that obtained with pneumoperitoneum.
- There is greater postoperative pain than with tension pneumo-peritoneum.

Because the physiological effects of pneumoperitoneum appear to be most marked after initial abdominal insufflation and during high pressure insufflation (> 14 mmHg), the use of a hybrid system of low pressure pneumoperitoneum (< 8 mmHg) combined with an abdominal wall retracting technique may provide the best of both worlds.

Pneumoperitoneum by Veress needle

Although the Veress needle remains in widespread use, open cannulation by the technique of Hasson or Fielding is our preferred method for inducing a pneumoperitoneum especially in a scarred abdomen. However, safe use of the Veress needle is as follows.

Unscarred abdomen

Site

- The Veress needle is most often inserted at the site where the primary 'laparoscope' cannula will be sited.

- The most common site entry is usually through, just above, or just below the umbilicus (Fig. 15). This is because the abdominal wall is thinnest at this point and is a relatively bloodless area. Contraindications to the use of the umbilical site include mid abdominal scar, portal hypertension, abnormal umbilicus, e.g. hernia or patent ductus or urachus.
- Other sites of entry involve pararectal lines in left upper or right lower quadrants (Fig. 15), and in female patients transuterine (fundal) or posterior fornix approaches may be used. Be aware of the liver in right upper quadrant, the common colonic adhesions in left lower quadrant and falciform ligament and bladder along the linea alba.
- There should be no hesitation in choosing a different site if adhesions, tissue mass or abnormal anatomy are suspected.

Technique

Hold the needle by the stem at about 2–4cm (depending on the thickness of the abdominal wall) from the tip with the thumb and forefinger (Fig. 16). For infra-umbilical entry (Fig. 17), grasp the full thickness of the abdominal wall (difficult in obese patients) just below the umbilicus.

Alternatively, with an assistant, one hand or a towel clip may be placed on each side of the lower margin of the umbilicus. This manoeuvre stabilizes the abdominal wall, provides a counter traction

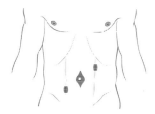

Fig. 15 The most common sites of entry for Veress needle in an unscarred abdomen.

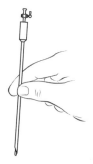

Fig. 16 Holding the Veress needle.

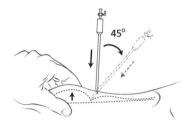

(a)

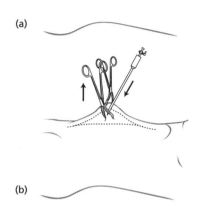

(b)

Fig. 17 Technique of insertion of the Veress needle for infra-umbilical entry. Hand (a) or towel clips (b) provide upward counter traction against the needle which is inserted first perpendicularly into the linea alba and then at 45° into the peritoneal cavity.

against the needle, and allows the bowel to fall away from the site of entry. Introduce the needle towards the centre of the pelvic cavity through a small stab incision using pressure from the wrist only. A rotatory movement may facilitate penetration. Resistance followed by a definite give with a click is usually experienced as the needle passes through the parietal peritoneum. Failure to hear a click may mean that the needle is faulty or has not penetrated the peritoneal layer. A 'give' may also be felt at the fascial level. Once the needle is in the correct place, its movement should be minimized to prevent complications of displacement and injury to the viscera.

Safety checks

A variety of tests are carried out to ensure that the needle is placed in the peritoneal cavity proper (Fig. 18):
• Free movement test: the tip of the needle should move freely from side to side. Any resistance may indicate that the needle is in a peri-peritoneal space or a peritoneal structure.
• Syringe test: a 5–10 ml syringe attached to the needle.
   (a) Aspirate for blood and visceral contents (bowel contents, bile, urine).

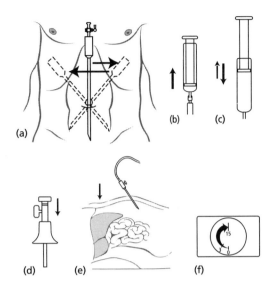

Fig. 18 Safety checks: (a) free movements; (b) aspiration with syringe; (c) instillation of 5–10 ml saline followed by aspiration; (d) saline meniscus rapidly descending within the needle; (e) percussion—liver dullness gradually disappearing; (f) insufflation pressure gradually rising.

(b) Gently instill 5–10 ml saline which should flow without resistance and not come back on aspiration. If some saline comes back the needle may still be extraperitoneal.

(c) If any saline is left in the hub of the needle this will be rapidly sucked into the peritoneal cavity when the abdominal wall is lifted.

• Insufflation test: The needle is attached to the gas tube, and a properly functioning and set insufflator (initial flow 1 l/min for adults, 100–500 ml/min for children; pressure 10–15 mmHg for adults, 6–10 mmHg for children) should give an initial pressure reading of 0–3 mmHg and rise gradually to its preset values. Incorrect placing of the needle is evident if the initial pressure is high and the flow is low.

• Percussion test: throughout the insufflation, make sure that the abdomen expands symmetrically and the insufflation is not confined to one region. Asymmetrical expansion may indicate either an extraperitoneal needle or intra-abdominal adhesions.

Insufflation

A rapid expansion (insufflation) of the peritoneal cavity may cause peri-operative cardiac dysrhythmias and postoperative pain and nausea. Therefore, the initial pneumoperitoneum should be established gradually to the required level of pressure with low gas flow (1 l/min adult, 100–500 ml/min paediatric). An established pneumoperitoneum requires 3–5 L of gas (450 mL–3 l in paediatrics). The gas flow may then be increased to 3–6 l/min (if possible keep below 1 l/min in paediatrics) so that an adequate pneumoperitoneum to the desired level of pressure is maintained (adult < 15 mmHg, paediatrics < 10 mmHg).

Throughout the entire insufflation process, the patient's ventilation, pulse, and blood pressure are monitored closely to ensure that complications are avoided.

Scarred abdomen

Special precautions are necessary to avoid damaging any adherent bowel.
• The history of the previous pathology and/or surgery may indicate the potential severity of the internal adhesions.
• Pre- or per-operative ultrasound scanning of the abdomen helps to localize the adhesions.
• Try the needle several centimetres away from the scar, for example: left upper quadrant or above umbilicus for lower abdominal scar; right lower quadrant or below umbilicus for upper abdominal scar (Fig. 19).
• The safety tests are carried out thoroughly.
• In difficult cases convert to open laparoscopy.

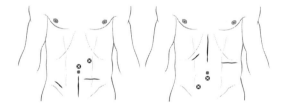

Fig. 19 Sites for Veress needle insertion in a scarred abdomen.

Problems and solutions of Veress needle and pneumoperitoneum

Misplaced Veress needle (Fig. 20) is the commonest source of complications in laparoscopy and rarely causes significant problems unless the gas flow is commenced.

Misplaced needle with or without insufflation

Subcutaneous fat:
  • Happens in the obese and results from oblique insertion of needle;
  • Often fails safety tests;

- If connected to gas flow, localized emphysema with a crackling feel develops;
- Reposition the needle, emphysema resolves spontaneously.

Extraperitoneal space:

- Relatively common especially in obese patients, with oblique insertion of needle, and in the lower abdomen;
- Often fails safety tests;
- If connected to gas flow emphysema develops;
- Reposition the needle. Emphysema may prevent or complicate repositioning of the needle.

Omentum:

- Fairly common especially in the obese;
- Often fails safety tests;
- Needle may cause haematoma formation;
- Needle and insufflation cause omental emphysema;
- Attempt to reposition the needle;
- Haematoma or emphysema may complicate the subsequent laparoscopic procedure.

Mesentery:

- Rare but potentially serious;
- Fails safety tests;
- Needle may cause haematoma or active bleed (rarely significant);

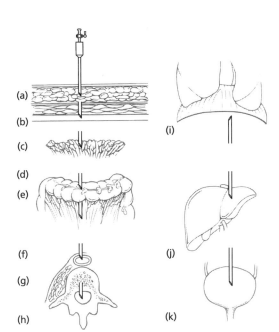

Fig. 20 Misplaced Veress needle. (a) Subcutaneous fat; (b) extraperitoneal space; (c) omentum; (d) intestine/ stomach; (e) mesentery/its vessels; (f) major vessels; (g) retroperitoneal space; (h) spine; (i) diaphragm/lung/pericardium; (j) liver/spleen/kidney; (k) bladder/ureters, uterus.

- Needle and insufflation produce emphysema, or gas embolus if in vessel;
- Attempt to reposition needle (except in hypotension and gas embolus where immediate resuscitation measures are required);
- Haematoma, emphysema and bleeding may complicate the subsequent laparoscopic procedure.

Small intestine, colon, stomach or bladder:
- Rare but potentially dangerous;
- Syringe aspiration produces contents;
- Reposition needle;
- Puncture site usually seals off spontaneously;
- Late peritonitis from missed perforation of gastrointestinal tract by Veress needle is very rare, but serious;

Liver, spleen, kidney and uterus:
- Rare but potentially serious;
- Often fails safety tests;
- Needle causes haematoma or active bleed (rarely significant);
- Needle and insufflation may lead to embolus;
- Attempt to reposition needle (except in gas embolus, hypotension and significant bleed where immediate treatment measures are required).

Major retroperitoneal vessel:
- Rare but potentially very dangerous;
- Syringe test aspirate blood;
- Needle penetration alone may result in small to medium haematoma, or expanding haematoma which indicates significant vascular injury. However, the needle may tear the inferior vena cava (IVC) resulting in massive haemorrhage;
- Needle and insufflation cause gas embolus;
- Reposition needle only if the surgeon is an experienced laparoscopist and there is no sign of expanding haematoma or embolus.

Diaphragm, heart and spine: very rare but potentially serious. An improperly placed Veress needle may be repositioned (except in expanding haematoma, significant bleed or gas embolus) following a partial or complete withdrawal and by reinsertion of the needle in a different direction or in a completely new site. Once a pneumoperitoneum is successfully created, a thorough examination of the suspected injured intra- or retroperitoneal structure is important. Perforation of intestinal tract and small bleed can successfully be controlled via a laparoscope. Any significant injury, however, must be dealt with via an immediate laparotomy.

Complications of pneumoperitoneum

See Physiological (page 9) and Pneumoperitoneum (page 30)
Major gas embolus:
- Extremely rare;
- Occurs with or without a vascular injury (direct vessel, liver, spleen, uterus, kidney);
- Low venous pressure facilitates gas embolus;
- Signs include sudden fall in end tidal CO_2 caused by sudden fall in lung perfusion and circulatory collapse;
- Management should consist of general resuscitation measures including, discontinuation of gas flow and desufflation, head down tilt, attempt to aspirate gas, and intravenous fluid;
- Watch for signs of active bleeding from the initial injury (syringe aspirate blood, expanding haematoma, hypotension) and deal with it accordingly.

Cardiac arrythmia:
- Relatively common especially in elderly and those with pre-existing illnesses;
- May occur as a result of hypoxia associated with inadequate ventilation or hypotension;
- Other causes include direct and rapid stretching of the peritoneum, vasovagal reflex or CO_2 irritation.

Hypotension:
- Rare;
- May result from reduced venous return, other complications or cardiac dysrhythmias;
- gas embolism and hypoxia;
- May be a feature of a pre-existing pathology or laparoscopic trauma.

Hypoxia.
Pneumothorax.
Subcutaneous emphysema of the head and neck, or genitalia and retroperitoneal or mediastinal emphysema without a direct needle puncture are not uncommon findings and may occur from gas tracking along the tissue planes. All resolve spontaneously over a short period of time.

Primary cannula insertion (1st cannula)

The most common cannula/trocar used is of 10–11 mm diameter with a safety shield/device. Larger cannulae allow a better gas flow when a 10mm scope is *in situ*. The usual site for the initial 'primary' cannula is the immediate subumbilical or supraumbilical region; remember that in obese and some times very old patients the umbilicus is positioned lower than normal.

The peri-umbilical route is preferred because:
- The abdominal wall is the thinnest.
- This region is relatively bloodless.
- It is a neutral site for the use of telescopes and instruments in most surgical procedures.
- The scar is cosmetically acceptable, particularly when the incision is placed circumferentially with the umbilical crease.

The contraindications to a peri-umbilical route are:
- Mid abdominal scar. (This is only a relative contraindication if the open cannulation technique is employed.)
- Abnormal umbilicus (hernia or remnant of ductus).
- Portal hypertension.

Most surgeons prefer a direct route for insertion of the cannula rather than the Z route (Fig. 21). The latter produces an indirect route, thereby reducing the chances of gas leak pre-operatively and hernia formation postoperatively. However, it is more difficult to use for replacing the cannula, and to dilate for retrieving organs such as the gall bladder. A Z route tends to keep the cannula in one direction which can be awkward to steer.

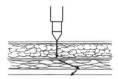

Fig. 21 The Z-route for cannula/trocar insertion.

Technique

After creation of the pneumoperitoneum, an adequate skin incision with a small nick in the linea alba is required. An assembled cannula and trocar is held firmly in the palm with the index or middle finger, extended along side the cannula to act as a brake 2–4 cm (depending on the size of the patient) from the tip of the trocar (Fig. 22a). As for insertion of the Veress needle, the subumbilical region is held firmly by the surgeons, or with an assistant, one hand or towel clip on each side of the lower margin of the umbilicus. The cannula/trocar are

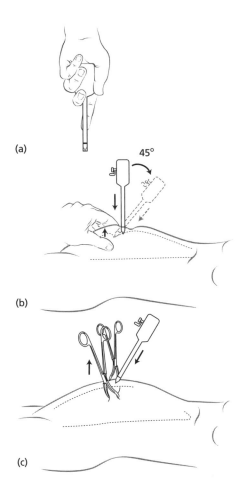

Fig. 22 Technique of insertion of the primary cannula/trocar for infraumbilical entry. (a) Holding the cannula/trocar; (b) hand; or (c) towel clips provide an upward counter-traction against the cannula/trocar which are inserted first perpendicularly into the linea alba and then at 45° into the peritoneal cavity.

introduced using continuous pressure with gentle twisting movement, initially perpendicular, and once the linea alba is engaged the tip is pointed towards the mid pelvis. (Remember that in obese patients, the umbilicus is positioned lower than normal; Fig. 22b,c.) A give with the click of the spring loaded safety shield/device indicates that the trocar is sufficiently advanced. In cannulae without a safety device, a give with a hissing sound of the gas escaping from the perforation near the tip of the trocar indicates that the peritoneum is breached. At this point, the trocar is withdrawn slightly, the cannula is advanced 1 or 2 cm and then the trocar is removed. There should be a whooshing sound of gas escaping through the cannula. At this stage, the cannula may be fixed if there is a grip on fixing device, and the position of the cannula is checked by the telescope/camera before the gas line is connected.

Primary cannula in the scarred abdomen

Once the pneumoperitoneum is established, the primary cannula/ trocar may be inserted where the greatest gas space is expected. A small cannula (5 mm) with a safety device may be easier to insert first. This will allow initial visualization and assessment of the peritoneal cavity by a 5 mm telescope if available. Larger cannulae (10–11 mm) can then be placed under direct internal vision or alternatively the small cannula replaced by a larger cannula (page 45). In difficult cases, the open technique of laparoscopy should be employed.

Problems and solutions of primary cannulae

The blind insertion of the primary cannula/trocar is by far the most dangerous step in any laparoscopic procedure even if there is an already established pneumoperitoneum. Do not insufflate through the primary cannula unless you are certain of the position or have first inspected the peritoneal cavity with a telescope.

Subcutaneous or extraperitoneal cannulation (Fig. 23)

• Extraperitoneal position is commoner because of the loose attachment, of the peritoneum, particularly in the lower abdomen.
• Occurs more often in obese or during oblique route insertion.
• Strands of tissue and fat are seen instead of bowel through telescope.
• May be prevented if an adequate skin incision and a small fascial nick are made, a more direct/perpendicular route of insertion is chosen (particularly in obese) and no change of direction until the fascial layer is almost penetrated.

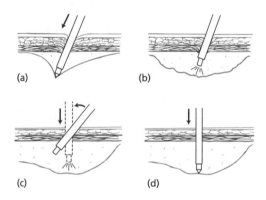

(a)   (b)
(c)   (d)

Fig. 23 Cannula in extraperitoneal space. (a) Peritoneum moves ahead of the trocar; (b) strands of tissue/fat are seen through the telescope; (c) direct the cannula under vision in a more perpendicular manner towards the peritoneal cavity; (d) replace the trocar and repass through the peritoneum.

- To reposition, insert the telescope inside the cannula, direct the cannula towards the peritoneal cavity in a more perpendicular position, and then exchange the telescope for the trocar and try to re pass the cannula/trocar once again.

Abdominal wall bleed (Fig. 34 on page 54)

- Common but usually minor.
- Significant bleed comes from the deep epigastric vessels.
- Not apparent without a telescope in peritoneal cavity.
- The bleed is usually a trickle which runs down the cannula and may disturb subsequent laparoscopic viewing.
- Significant bleed may be stopped, but only when secondary cannulae are in place (page 52).
- Prevent by placing your port in a known avascular site.

Omental injury

- Lobules of omental fat are seen through the telescope.
- Minor active bleeding or haematoma may occur as the cannula is gently removed.
- May complicate subsequent laparoscopic procedure.
- Once the secondary cannulae are in place, carefully examine and treat appropriately.

Mesentery injury

- Usually a haematoma which requires no active treatment.
- An active bleed, though rare, may complicate the subsequent laparoscopic procedure, and be potentially dangerous.
- Once the secondary cannulae are in place, a thorough assessment may reveal the extent of the injury.
- A laparoscopic ligature, stitch, clip or diathermy may stop most bleeds.
- Rarely, a major bleed may have to be dealt with via a formal laparotomy.

Injury to bowel, stomach or bladder

- Rare, but potentially lethal.
- May be just a serosal tear or haematoma, in which case no action is required.
- The inside or mucosal layer of the injured hollow viscus may be

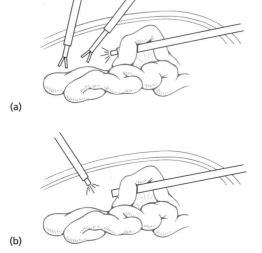

(a)

(b)

Fig. 24 Through and through intestinal/mesenteric injury by the primary cannula/trocar. (a) Telescope through the primary cannula fails to recognize the injury; (b) telescope through a secondary cannula may recognize the injury.

seen via the telescope in complete injury.
• Withdraw the cannula/telescope, and once the secondary cannulae are in place, a thorough examination of the injured site is mandatory.
• Through and through injury, a rare occurrence, may fail to be recognized unless you routinely inspect the site of the primary cannula through a secondary cannula (Fig. 24).
• All penetration injuries to a viscus must be repaired either laparoscopically or via a laparotomy, using stitches, endoloops, clips or a combination.
• Late peritonitis (few days postoperative) may occur if the perforation is missed.

Injury to major retroperitoneal vessels

• Tay cause immediate death.
• Three situations may arise: blood immediately fills or shoots out of the cannula, leave the cannula in place to tamponade; an expanding haematoma is seen through the telescope; blood rapidly fills the peritoneal cavity.
• Immediately cease insufflation but do not desufflate completely as this facilitates rapid laparotomy (remember gas embolus in venous injury). Tip the head of the table down, keep the venous pressure high, and proceed with laparotomy while asking for more blood and a more experienced surgeon or even a vascular surgeon.

- At laparotomy, immediate pressure should be applied and a quick and careful search is made to examine the extent of the injury.

Injury to liver, spleen and kidney

- Potentially serious.
- Blood may or may not fill the cannula.

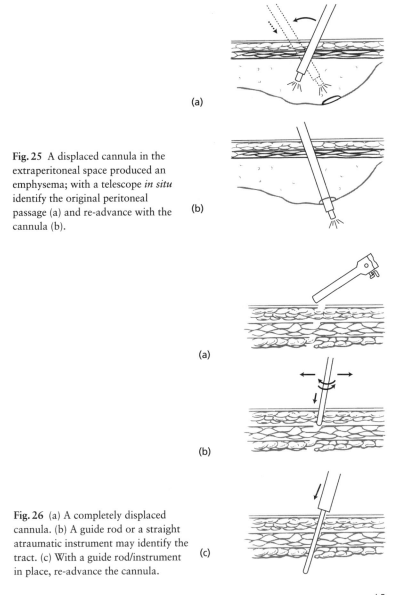

(a)

Fig. 25 A displaced cannula in the extraperitoneal space produced an emphysema; with a telescope *in situ* identify the original peritoneal passage (a) and re-advance with the cannula (b).

(b)

(a)

(b)

Fig. 26 (a) A completely displaced cannula. (b) A guide rod or a straight atraumatic instrument may identify the tract. (c) With a guide rod/instrument in place, re-advance the cannula.

(c)

- Active bleeding from solid organs must be assessed thoroughly via the laparoscope or laparotomy, and preferably managed conservatively unless proved otherwise.
- A constant trickle of blood may seriously jeopardize any subsequent laparoscopic procedure. Blood absorbs light and reduces visibility in the laparoscopic operating field.
- Remember gas embolus.

Injury to ureters

- Very rare.
- Partial or complete, requires immediate attention.

Partial displacement of the cannula (Fig. 25)

- Extraperitoneal emphysema may develop.
- With the telescope in place, re-advance the cannula under direct vision.

Complete displacement of the cannula (Fig. 26)

- With the telescope inside the cannula, re-advance the cannula under vision.
- Or replace the trocar and re-advance the cannula.
- Or place a guide rod/straight blunt instrument through the track and re-advance the cannula with or without the gradual dilator system.

Gas leak (see page 54), *problems with imaging* (see page 20)

Open cannulation (Hasson's technique)

Blind insertion of the Veress needle and/or the primary cannula may cause:
- Injury to the viscera and vessels which are rare, but can be serious.
- Extraperitoneal gas insufflation which is relatively common but causes little harm.

The technique of open laparoscopy provides an alternative and relatively safe method especially in the scarred abdomen, for insertion of the primary cannula and creation of a pneumoperitoneum. Overall, the technique is not slower than that of blind insertion of the cannula as positioning of the most important cannula and subsequent closure of the defect are made much easier. The procedure entails surgical exposure of the peritoneal cavity via an incision where the primary cannula is usually placed (sites discussed previously for the blind primary cannula, page 39) using either a modified Hasson's cannula or an ordinary cannula. The incision has to be large enough, particularly in the obese, to allow safe exposure and application of the anchoring sutures or purse-string. Where abdominal scarring exists from previous surgery, the incision may be placed elsewhere in the abdominal wall as for the blind technique.

The modified Hasson's cannula has an outer sliding conical flange to maintain the seal at the site of entry and prevent the cannula from falling to the peritoneal cavity. It also has struts on either side for anchoring sutures to prevent the cannula from falling out, and a blunt trocar (Fig. 27).

An ordinary cannula requires one or two towel clips or an anchoring sleeve (spiral retaining collar) to keep the cannula in place and prevent gas leak (Fig. 28). It is a simple and effective technique but there is a slight tendency for the cannula to displace inwards and outwards. Alternatively a purse string suture or a single stitch with a single throw around the cannula which is then tied to the gas port, may be used to prevent gas leak and outwards displacement (Fig. 29). The anchoring stitch/purse-string also allows tenting of the anterior abdominal wall to facilitate low pressure laparoscopy and safe and easy closure of the fascial wound at the end of the procedure.

Struts
Suture
Screw to fix the conical flange
Outer sliding conical flange

Fig. 27 A modified Hasson's cannula in place.

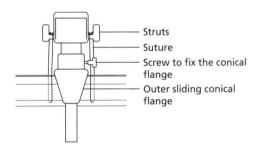

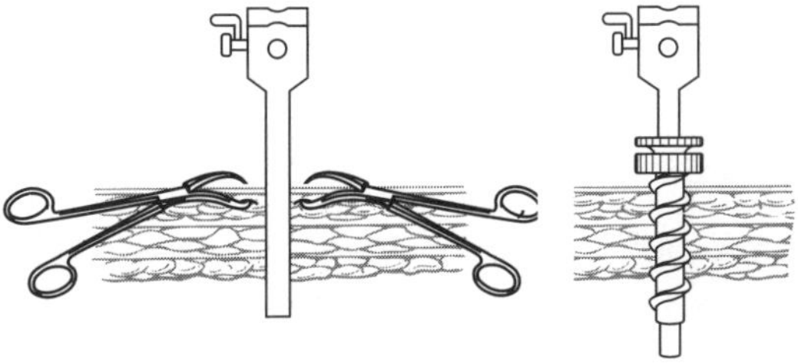

Fig. 28 An ordinary cannula requires one or two towel clips or an anchoring sleeve to keep the cannula in place and prevent gas leak.

47

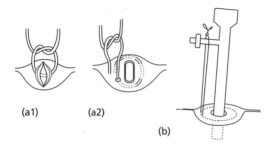

(a1)   (a2)

(b)

Fig. 29 Open cannulation with an ordinary cannula and an anchoring suture. (a1/a2) A single suture or a purse-string through fascia and peritoneum to prevent outwards displacement, and a single throw to prevent gas leak. (b) Cannula in place.

Complications of the open technique

• The technique is more difficult in obese patients because of the depth of subcutaneous fat and excessive extraperitoneal fat.
• There is a potential for bowel injury where adhesions exist near or at the incision site.
• Cannula displacement may occur if the anchoring or purse-string sutures are not properly secured.

Secondary cannula (working cannula, accessory cannula)

While some diagnostic laparoscopy is achievable via a single primary cannula, the vast majority of laparoscopic procedures require one to five secondary 'working cannulae'.

Selection

These may be reusable or disposable, with or without a proper valve and/or safety shield/device, though membrane gas sealant around the instrument is essential. At least one of the secondary cannulae should have a side gas port. This provides an additional gas port and allows the gas line (tube) to be moved away from the telescope cannula when needed as in cases of fogging of telescope or insufficient gas flow because of an inadequate space within the telescope cannula (10mm telescope in 10.5 mm cannula).

The size and length of these secondary cannulae depend on the patient and the type of procedure to be performed.

Position

The position of the secondary cannula depends on the type of surgery to be executed and the following rules help to facilitate access (Fig. 30):

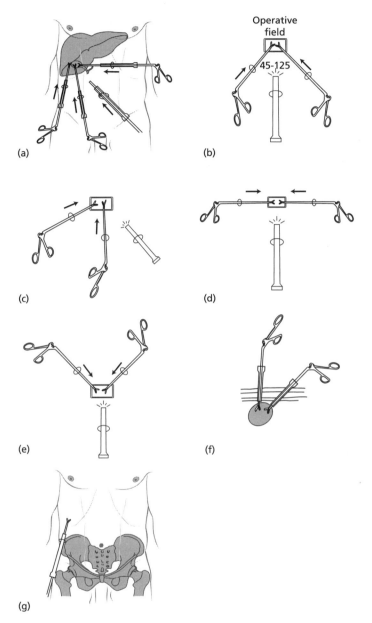

Fig. 30 Position of secondary cannulae. (a) All cannulae directed towards the operating field; (b,c) cannulae in front and sides of the telescope; (d) straight line instruments; (e) instruments against the line of view; (f) cannula close to operative field; (g) cannula close to bone.

- Mark the sites after the creation of the pneumoperitoneum.
- The direction of insertion should be towards the operative field. Other directions result in difficulty delivering the hand instruments to the operative field.
- Secondary cannulae are best sited on either side and in front of the telescope to facilitate hand–eye co-ordination and to keep the working instruments in view.
- Keep any two working cannulae at 45–125° angle if possible (optimal 65°) in order to:

    (a) Facilitate working with instruments;

    (b) Minimize cannula and instrument clash at the surface and inside the abdomen.

- Straight line instruments are difficult to manoeuvre. Instruments entering the abdomen against the line of view give mirror imaging, consequently they are extremely difficult to operate.
- Avoid placing the cannulae too close to the operative field as there will be insufficient room for the grasper or scissors jaws to operate.
- Avoid placing the cannulae too close to bony landmarks, as hard fixed structure such as bones restrict free cannula/instrument movements.

Technique

The size of the skin incision should be equal to that of the cannula (10 mm incision for 10 mm cannula). A small nick in the fascia may facilitate insertion of cannulae larger than 5 mm. As for insertion of the primary cannula an assembled cannula and trocar is held firmly with the index or middle finger acting as a stop. Under direct telescopic view the cannula/trocar is introduced using continuous pressure with gentle twisting movement, initially perpendicular, and once the fascia/muscle is engaged, the tip is directed towards the operative field. Peritoneal movement ahead of the trocar is more likely with oblique routes (Fig. 31). In obese patients the route of entry may have to be directly perpendicular.

If the tip of the trocar approaches too close to the underlying viscera one or more of the following may be required:

- Lift up the abdominal wall by hand or towel clips against the

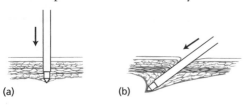

(a)   (b)

Fig. 31 Insertion of cannula. First perpendicular (a) then oblique (b). Note the peritoneal movement ahead of the trocar in the oblique route.

line of cannula/trocar penetration (Fig. 32a).

- Increase pressure of the pneumoperitoneum.
- Once the tip of the trocar is seen behind the peritoneum, the direction of insertion of the cannula is changed away from the viscera (Fig. 32b). To avoid internal injury, the cannula/trocar may have to be inserted parallel to the abdominal wall (Fig. 32c), or in the direction of the telescope or even directly into the primary cannula. In the latter two situations, the telescope must be withdrawn well into the cannula in order to avoid damaging the telescope (Fig. 32d).
- If other cannulae are in place, counter traction may be applied by a direct drive into the cannula, or an instrument inserted via the existing cannula which may facilitate the entry of another cannula (Fig. 33b–d).

Once the secondary cannulae are in place, the position of the primary cannula which has been inserted blindly may be checked by a telescope through a secondary cannula.

Problems and solutions

Peritoneal movement ahead of the trocar

- More likely with oblique route of entry (Fig. 31), lower abdominal insertion caused by loosely attached peritoneum, and in children.

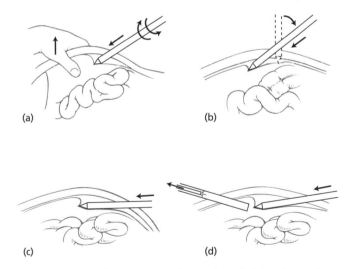

(a) (b)

(c) (d)

Fig. 32 The site of cannula insertion too close to the underlying viscera. Arrows indicate direction of movement/pressure. (a) Lift the abdominal wall; (b) change of direction; (c) insertion parallel to the abdominal wall and viscera; (d) direction towards/into the telescope cannula with the telescope being withdrawn into the cannula.

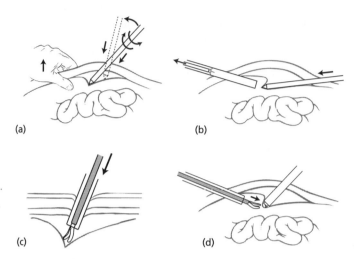

Fig. 33 Peritoneal movement ahead of the trocar. (a) Stabilize the abdominal wall by hand or towel clips; (b) direct the trocar into the primary cannula with the telescope being withdrawn; (c) cut the peritoneum with an instrument inside the cannula; (d) counter-traction against the incoming cannula by another cannula or an instrument, or cut the overlying peritoneum.

• Try to stabilize the abdominal wall by grasping it with hand or towel clips, direct the cannula/trocar more perpendiculaly, and exert slight twisting movement (Fig. 33a).
• Direct the cannula/trocar into the primary port with the telescope being withdrawn sufficiently to avoid damage (Fig. 33b).
• Remove the trocar and try to cut the peritoneum with a sharp instrument inserted through the cannula (Fig. 33c).
• If other secondary cannulae are in place, exert counter traction against the incoming cannula/trocar or direct the incoming cannula/trocar into it, or use an instrument through the existing cannula to cut the peritoneum ahead of the incoming cannula (Fig. 33d).

Prematurely activated safety shield/device

• May happen at any time during the passage of the cannula/trocar, caused either by a relaxed grip on the trocar, or when the system reaches a low resistance plane of tissue as in the extraperitoneal space.
• Rearm by resetting the trocar and keep a firm grip on the system. Occasionally a slight change of direction may help.
• Sometimes, an instrument inserted through the cannula or another cannula may have to be used to cut through the peritoneum to allow the incoming cannula to pass through (Fig. 33c–d).

Safety shield not springing

This is usually caused by too small a skin incision which prevents the shield from advancing.

Injury to viscera and major vessels. As for primary cannula (page 39).

Abdominal wall haemorrhage (Fig. 34)

• Usually minor, but significant haemorrhage from deep epigastric vessels may cause problems.
• Some vessels are recognized, by transilluminating the abdominal wall using the laparoscope light within, or by focusing the laparoscope onto known anatomical landmarks such as deep epigastric vessels.
• Press the cannula in the direction of the bleed. This may be sufficient to stop the bleeding.
• Continuous significant bleeding can be stopped by intracorporal suture ligature; percutaneous suture ligature in thin or paediatric cases; percutaneously inserted straight needle with suture in large or obese patients; or by percutaneously inserted suture through a suture holder. Absorbable sutures are cut flush on the skin, while non-absorbable sutures are easily removed after 12–24 h. Alternatively, a Foley's catheter may be inserted through the cannula site, the balloon inflated and traction exerted until the bleeding stops.

Significant bleed from unknown origin

• A thorough check of all organs and possible locations is required to find and treat the source.
• Remember other sources of bleeding: operative field, instrument and retractor injury, adhesiolysis, etc.

Cannula dislodgement

• Anchoring devices (Fig. 13, page 29) may not always prevent this happening.
• Replace the trocar and re-advance the cannula.
• A guide rod/straight instrument may facilitate replacement (Figs. 25 and 26, page 45).

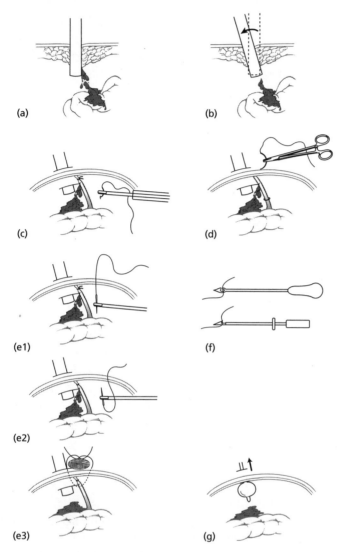

Fig. 34 Abdominal wall haemorrhage from cannula insertion. (a) Significant bleed; (b) press the cannula against the bleed; (c and d) intracorporeal or percutaneous suture ligature to stop the bleeding; (e1–3) percutaneously inserted and intracorporeally assisted suture ligature over a roll of gauze; (f) suture holder; (g) Foley's catheter stops bleeding.

Gas leak and/or loss of pneumoperitoneum

- Ensure gas supply is adequate.
- Ensure all connections are tight: insufflator to gas line, gas line to cannula, parts of the assembled cannula if reusable.
- Ensure gas ports on non-insufflating cannulae are closed.

- Examine for faulty valve, diaphragm, or rubber gas sealant.
- Large incision around cannula. Here a single suture or purse-string suture to include all abdominal wall layers may stop gas leakage. Otherwise a grip on the anchoring device, replacement for a larger diameter cannula, or suturing the incision and replacing the cannula in another site may be required.
- Displaced cannulae should be re-sited.
- Instruments, or reducer may be mismatched.

Adhesions

Adhesiolysis may be necessary to create room for placing secondary cannulae.

Retraction

Appropriate retraction is an essential component of any laparoscopic exposure, and may be achieved by the following means.

Gravity

Appropriate positioning of the patient, such as Trendelenburg, reverse Trendelenburg, or lateral rotation, may all allow peritoneal structures to fall away from the operative field.

Grasping forceps

Tissue planes may be revealed by traction or counter traction using any kind of grasping forceps.

Retractor

Specifically designed reusable or disposable instruments in varying sizes and shapes are available to use as retractors (Fig. 35). During retraction, grasping forceps and retractors can damage viscera, especially the liver, if not used with care. Retractor injuries may occur as a result of:
- Direct perforation by the instruments despite their blunt ends.
- Pressure splitting of liver, or tense distended loops of bowel.
- Direct or indirect coupling from the electrocoagulation heat energy.
- Fan retractors may trap and injure bowel or liver during their closure (Fig. 36).

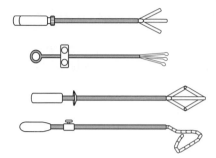

Fig. 35 Different types of retractors.

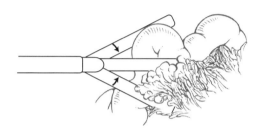

Fig. 36 Fan retractor may trap and damage viscera during closure.

Extraperitoneal laparoscopy

The routine use of the extraperitoneal approach in established open surgical procedures, such as hernia repair, urinary operations and ileofemoral vessel reconstruction, facilitates access and avoids the morbidity that may be associated with traversing the peritoneal cavity.

Extraperitonoscopy may be performed effectively within a space created by breaking up the connective tissue binding and the extraperitoneal space with either, direct CO_2 insufflation or a balloon dissector.

Current indications are:
- Herniotomy
- Nephrectomy
- Adrenalectomy
- Pyelolithotomy
- Pyeloplasty
- Ureterolithotomy
- Ligation of testicular veins for varicocele
- Pelvic lymphadenectomy
- Colposuspension
- Ileo femoral vascular reconstruction
- Lumbar sympathectomy.

Technique with balloon

A 1–2 cm skin incision is made at an infraumbilical position for hernia repair, varicocele ligation, colposuspension, pelvic lymph node and lower ureter; or just below the tip of the 12th rib or above and medial to the anterior superior iliac spine for renal and upper ureteric surgery. Blunt dissection is carried down to the preperitoneal plane. Using the index finger and/or a conventional artery forceps (usually a 2 cm skin and muscle incision is required) or a specifically designed space maker/cannula (1 cm incision is required) towards the operating field, a space is created for the balloon in the extraperitoneal plane (Fig. 37). The balloon dissector is then placed in the space and distended with 250–1500 ml of saline, depending on the size of the

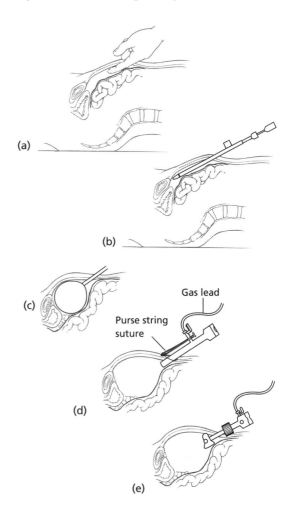

Fig. 37 Creation of a pneumoextraperitoneum. (a) Preperitoneal finger dissection; (b) space maker dissection; (c) balloon inflation to create space; (d) a purse-string suture to keep the cannula in position and prevent gas leak; (e) a specifically designed primary cannula for extraperitoneal laparoscopy (outside flange and inside balloon prevent the cannula from falling in and out, respectively).

patient and the nature of the operation to be performed. The balloon is left distended for a few to several minutes to achieve haemostasis, and it is then decompressed and removed. A reasonable, but less efficient, balloon dissector may be fashioned by tying a rubber glove over an 18F catheter.

A strong, absorbable purse-string suture is inserted through muscle/fascia, and an appropriately sized primary cannula is pushed over its trocar (or cannula with blunt trocar) through the purse-string into the extraperitoneal space and secured with a single throw of the suture, thus allowing snug opposition of the muscle/fascia to the cannula during the procedure and preventing gas leakage. The suture is then secured around the gas inlet (gas port) of the cannula, allowing 1 or 2 cm of the tip of the cannula to remain within the extraperitoneal space (Fig. 37d). An alternative to this technique of purse-stringing an ordinary cannula, a specifically designed disposable primary cannula may be used (Fig. 37e). The primary cannula is connected to the insufflator and a pneumoextraperitoneum is established and maintained at a pressure of 5–15 mmHg (a pressure of 8–10 mmHg is sufficient in most adults). At this point 2–4 L of gas should have been instilled.

The telescope is then inserted through the primary cannula, and after exploration of the cavity, the size and position of the secondary 'working' cannulae are selected based on the size of the patient and nature of the procedure to be performed.

Technique without balloon

The above procedure is repeated without the use of the balloon (incision, blunt dissection with finger and/or forceps, and purse-stringed cannula). A zero degree telescope is inserted into the preperitoneal plane via the cannula, and the cannula is then connected to the gas flow (pressure 6–10 mmHg). Under direct vision, the tip of the telescope and the force of the insufflation are used to break up the connective tissue binding the extraperitoneal space and a satisfactory pneumoextraperitoneum is created (Fig. 38).

Alternatively, some surgeons advocate using the Veress needle and direct CO_2 insufflation to create the initial extraperitoneal space. A primary cannula is then inserted via a stab incision.

Potential advantages

• Avoids the morbidity that may be associated with traversing the peritoneal cavity.

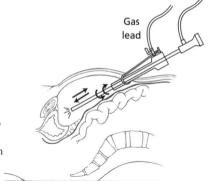

Fig. 38 Creation of a
pneumoextraperitoneum using the tip
of the telescope and the force of
insufflation. Arrows indicate direction
of force/movement used by the tip of
the telescope.

- Irrigation and suction of the space is rarely necessary.
- Allows surgery with relative ease in patients who have intra-peritoneal adhesions.

Disadvantages

- Contraindicated in patients with bleeding disorders, malignant conditions (except pelvic lymphadenectomy), and in previously scarred extraperitoneum.
- It has a limited value in obese, extraperitoneal fibrosis and paediatric patients.
- The effectiveness of dissection depends on the position of the balloon, cannula or Veress needle in the first place.
- During distension with the balloon, there is a tendency for the balloon to migrate towards the area of minimal resistance. Therefore, a second or specifically shaped balloon may be required to create the desired space.
- Peritoneal tear and extension pneumoperitoneum may occur at any stage of the procedure and make extraperitoneal surgery difficult to achieve.
- There is a potential for:
  (a) Gas embolus (use low pressure gas insufflation).
  (b) Avulsing vessels (e.g. spermatic, inferior mesenteric in retroperitoneal procedures).
  (c) Damaging the inferior vena cava and duodenum in right-sided retroperitonoscopy, and pancreas and colon on the left.
  (d) Surgical emphysema (subcutaneous, chest) which resolves spontaneously and rapidly.

Instrument holder

During laparoscopy, adequate and precise assistants are essential. Currently, most surgeons rely on trainee surgeons to hold the telescope, retractor and other instruments and it is not uncommon to have more than one assistant at the operating table. Any lack of experience or unfamiliarity with the use of laparoscopic telescopes and instruments can be frustrating or even dangerous. Additionally, during certain phases of many laparoscopic procedures, items such as the telescope and retractors may not have to be changed and could remain in a relatively fixed position for appreciable periods of time. Here, an instrument holder with adjustable arms and joint may prove beneficial. There are several different types of instrument holders available to use, but the ideal instrument holder should have the following characteristics:
- User friendly and causes no obstruction to the surgeon.
- Has a secure locking system and a universal instrument holding device.
- No limit to its positioning capacity.
- Partly or completely sterilizable and easily adjustable by a single hand or even a remote controller.

Exiting from the abdomen

- Depending on the type of laparoscopic procedure, suction and irrigation with or without antibiotics/antiseptic may be necessary to recheck for bleeding and remove clots, pus, debris and other fluids from the peritoneal cavity.
- Thoroughly inspect the operative field and the whole area around and in between access cannulae for bleeding, and signs of an inadvertent injury to vessels, and viscera and deal with it accordingly.
- Remove all working instruments under vision and ensure no omentum is drawn into cannula lumen.
- Check for signs of pericannular bleeding before and after removal of the cannula and deal with it accordingly.
   (a) A suture within or percutaneously or Foley's catheter as described previously (Fig. 34, page 54).
   (b) Or remove the cannula and apply a circular/or figure of eight suture through or around the skin incision.
   (c) In difficult cases, the wound may be enlarged and the bleeding point secured directly.
- Check and empty fluid/gas-filled hernia/hydrocele sac in male patients.

- Maintain a degree of pneumoperitoneum until the last cannula, and systematically remove the cannulae if possible, as follows.

  (a) First, remove large secondary cannula and close the fascia/muscle defect with absorbable sutures while watching through the telescope (Fig. 39).

  (b) Next remove the primary cannula (in blind technique laparoscopy or open technique without an anchoring suture), close the defect while observing through a small telescope via a small secondary cannula.

  (c) The primary cannula in open laparoscopy with anchoring/purse-string sutures is left to the end because the already existing sutures are used to close the defect.

  (d) Finally remove the smaller secondary cannulae (5mm cannulae in adults and 3.5 mm in children are safe not to close).

- The skin may be closed with interrupted, subcuticular sutures or Steri-strips. Dressings are not usually required.

- Remove nasogastric tube and urinary catheter if they were inserted.

Problems after exiting

- Unrecognized visceral injury, from trocar insertion, instrumentation and diathermy may present later with peritonitis, intra abdominal abscess or enterocutaneous fistula. This complication is very rare, but potentially lethal.

- Puncturing and suturing bowel to the wound during wound closure.

- Herniation of bowel or omentum through cannula sites. These may occur either immediately after laparoscopy or present late as an incisional hernia.

- Haematoma at cannula site.

- Acute scrotal swelling from communicating hydrocele can be very painful particularly if it contains infected fluid.

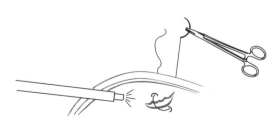

Fig. 39 Closure of large cannula wound under telescopic internal vision.

Instruments for dissection

Grasping forceps

Holding or grasping instruments are available in sizes, shapes and forms that suit different purposes. Generally, disposable instruments are less precise but lighter than reusable instruments. Newer, reusable instruments have been developed that allow dismantling for cleaning purposes, and changing parts rather than the whole instrument when necessary.

Tip/jaws (Fig. 40)

Single or double jaw mechanism. The latter allows larger grasp and blunt dissection.

Atraumatic or traumatic. All grasping forceps are traumatic to some extent. However, those with teeth or claws are obviously very traumatic. The more pointed or narrowed jaws are more traumatic, and some spring loaded forceps can be fairly traumatic.

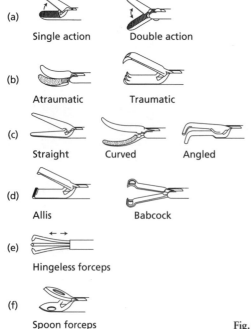

(a) Single action   Double action

(b) Atraumatic   Traumatic

(c) Straight   Curved   Angled

(d) Allis   Babcock

(e) Hingeless forceps

(f) Spoon forceps

Fig. 40 Grasping forceps—jaws.

Atraumatic, straight, curved or angled jaws (short or long). These are good for grasping, blunt dissection and suturing.

Allis and Babcock. These are fairly atraumatic holding devices.

Hingeless grasping forceps. Very traumatic but good for retrieving tissues or stones.

Spoon. This device is useful for biopsy or removal of small stones.

Handle (Fig. 41)

These come in different shapes, but most have a scissors type, angled or non-angled handle, which are good for grasping, blunt dissection and suturing. However, straight handles (non-scissors type) are only good for grasping and suturing.

Plain or self-holding (ratchet or spring loaded) the former is useful for all purposes, but the latter is only good for grasping. The ratchet handle is superior to the spring loaded handle. The former (ratchet) allows gentle adjustment at a fixed point, while the latter's function depends on the memory of the metal spring.

Shaft

• Available in length ranging from 20 to 50 cm and diameters 3–12 mm.
• Many are insulated with a terminal which can be connected to diathermy units.

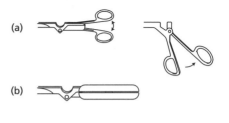

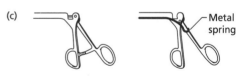

Fig. 41 Grasping forceps—handles.
(a) Scissors type straight and angled;
(b) straight non-scissors type; (c) self-holding ratchet and spring loaded.

- Light reflection from non-insulated instruments interferes with laparoscopic viewing.
- Some have a side port for flushing during cleaning.
- Most have rotating control to optimize the angle of use.

Scissors

Scissors are either disposable or reusable. Disposable scissors are less steady and less economical than reusable ones, but have the advantages of being sharp and absolutely sterile at all times.

Tips (jaws, blades) (Fig. 42)

Curved, double action jaw scissors. These are multipurpose but usually used for dissection with or without diathermy. To avoid accidental thermal injury to adjacent structures during diathermy dissection, especially in small operative spaces, the insulation sleeve should come right down to the moving blades (Fig. 42a).

Fine pointed, curved or straight microscissors. Usually used for microdissection or incisions into small structures such as the cystic duct or ureter.

Hooked scissors. These are appropriate for cutting ligated vessels, and other tubular structures, as well as ligatures. They prevent accidental damage to nearby structures by lifting away the structures to be cut. They also prevent tissues and ligatures from slipping out of the jaws.

Straight single or double jaw action with or without serration. These are useful to cut pedicles and sutures.

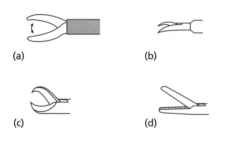

(a)

(b)

(c)

(d)

Fig. 42 Scissors—jaws. (a) Double action curved (note the insulation sleeve is down to the moving blades); (b) single action curved microscissors; (c) single action hooked; (d) single action straight.

Handle (Fig. 43)

Most have a scissor type, but angled handle. However, less popular straight handles are also available.

Fig. 43 Scissors—handles. (a) Ordinary handle with diathermy point; (b) straight.

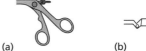

(a)   (b)

Shaft

• Available in lengths ranging from 20 to 50 cm and diameters 3–5 mm.
• Most are insulated so that they can be used with diathermy. However, they are rapidly blunted if used to cauterize tissue.
• Nearly all have rotating tips to maximize the angle of use.
• Many reusable scissors have a flushing port for cleaning. Others can be dismantled which allows easy cleaning, and part of the scissors, particularly the jaws which can be blunted, to be changed at a low cost. This particular characteristic renders the scissors less steady than they would be otherwise.

Diathermy/electrocautery

Electrocautery devices are widely available and familiar to all surgeons. Although monopolar coagulation or cutting currents are used commonly, bipolar coagulation is regarded as the safer option. Currently, bipolar cutting and electrohydrothermia systems are being developed, as are ultrasonic dissectors.

To achieve diathermy, a closed electrical circuit is necessary. In the case of the monopolar system, the current is applied through the electrode (live electrode), flows through the tissue to be coagulated or incised, then passes through the body and leaves via a large neutral pad (grounding pad) back into the generator. As biological tissue (patient's body) provides a much lower conductivity compared with the metallic wire and electrode of the diathermy system, and because the interface between the electrode and body tissue (surgical site) forms a small area of connection, the conversion of diathermy energy concentrates onto the small surgical site. This high concentration of energy results in coagulation or cutting of the surgical site (Fig. 44).

In the case of the bipolar system, both the active electrode (live electrode) and the neutral electrode (grounding pad) are built into the tip of the instrument. Thus, the interaction is restricted to the precise small area of tissue in between the two paths of the applied instrument (Fig. 45). The result is a safer interaction with a lower energy input.

With the monopolar system (Fig. 46), coagulation is best achieved by grasping the tissue with an insulated atraumatic forceps whilst the energy is delivered. Cutting is achieved by placing a fine electrode in such a way that it is just about to touch the surface to be incised.

In addition to the power used, the efficacy of coagulation or cutting is determined by the shape of the electrode. Hook, ball and the flat surface of a spatula are useful for coagulation, while needle, fine hook and edge of a spatula are suited to cutting (Fig. 47).

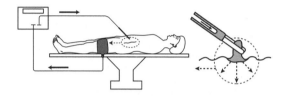

Fig. 44 Unipolar diathermy system. Energy passes through the body and leaves via neutral pad.

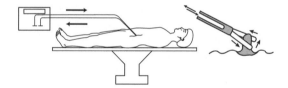

Fig. 45 Bipolar system. Energy passes in between the two blades only.

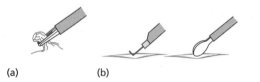

(a)   (b)

Fig. 46 Monopolar diathermy. (a) Coagulation using forceps; (b) cutting with hook or spatula.

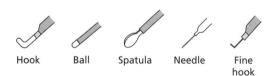

Hook   Ball   Spatula   Needle   Fine hook

Fig. 47 Diathermy probes.

With appropriate power setting, a semicircular or an L-shaped hook is one of the most useful devices for all purposes. It allows manipulation, blunt dissection, cutting and coagulation. Cutting may be achieved by either pulling or preferably using the heel of the hook (Fig. 48). In any case, care must be taken not to injure other tissues in the vicinity, particularly during pulling tissue out of the visual field (Fig. 49) when the tip of the electrode may hit another structure.

Precautions, problems and solutions of diathermy

• Before starting any laparoscopic procedure, make sure that the diathermy machine, cables and instrument terminals are compatible.
• Because diathermy produces high frequency signals, close proximity to video equipment can lead to interference on the monitor. Therefore, keep the diathermy cable separate from that of the camera, and try not to plug both instruments into the same mains supply.
• To avoid accidental burns from current leakage, check that the insulation sleeves of all instruments and cables are intact.
• As a rule of thumb:
  (a) The power setting should be minimum.
  (b) Never activate the diathermy prior to contact of the electrode with the tissue.
  (c) Activate the electrode for a minimum required duration at any one time.

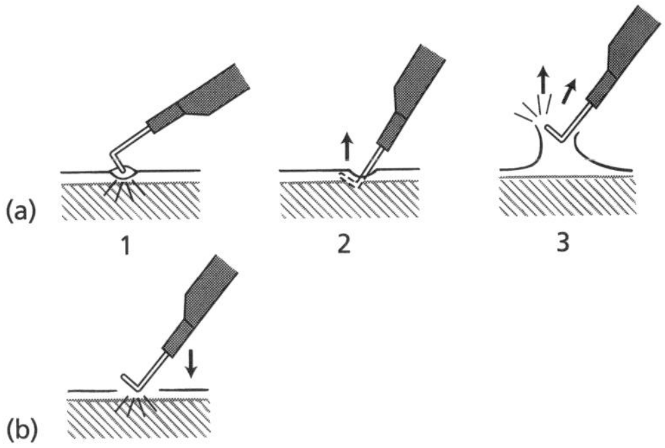

Fig. 48 Cutting with monopolar diathermy using a hook: (a, 1–3) by pulling; (b) with the heel of the hook.

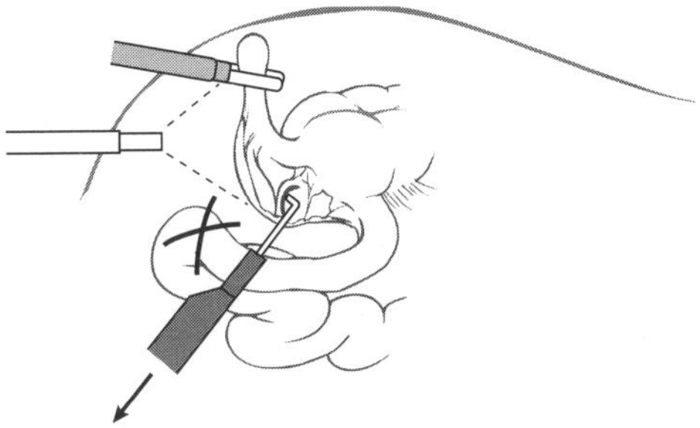

Fig. 49 Electrothermal injury to viscera during pulling technique diathermy.

(d) Always keep the uninsulated tip of the electrode in the viewing field.

• After each use, for a few seconds, the tip of the activated electrode remains very hot. Therefore avoid using the instrument for manipulating or touching other tissues immediately after use.

• Smoke may be eliminated from the peritoneal cavity by intermittent desufflation and insufflation.

• During monopolar coagulation a high density current conversion may take place at a nearby constricted small tissue area other than the surgical contact site. This may result in an unnoticed burn point which may then cause bleeding or peritonitis some time after laparoscopy. The examples are: tied base of appendix, tied cystic duct or any tied vessel or pedicle (Fig. 50).

• Direct coupling may occur if a monopolar active electrode accidentally touches an uninsulated (conductive) metal instrument, telescope or cannula (second conductor) (Fig. 51a). This action allows the second conductor to act as an active electrode and may cause and electrothermal injury in or beyond the viewing field.

• Sometimes an active monopolar electrode induces an unintended

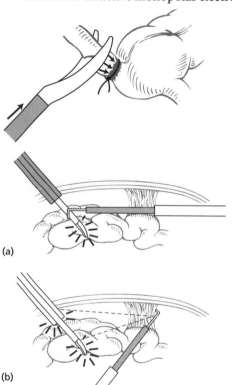

Fig. 50 Transecting appendix with an active diathermy scissors may allow electrothermal energy transfer to the tied base of appendix, thereby causing burn injury to the base of appendix and caecal wall.

(a)

(b)

Fig. 51 Monopolar diathermy injury. (a) Direct coupling; (b) indirect (capacitive) coupling with instrument or cannula.

or stray current into a nearby uninsulated (conductive) or partly insulated instrument, telescope, or cannula. This effect is termed 'capacitive coupling' or 'indirect coupling'. Under certain conditions, this unintended current on the second conductor can cause sparks and burns (Fig. 51b). Unfortunately, as in direct coupling, these types of injuries usually occur outside the surgeon's view.

• A combination of metal cannula (conductor) and plastic anchoring device (non-conductor) which prevents dissipation of energy from the metal to the abdominal wall is an ideal situation for indirect coupling. This combination should therefore never be used, but instead either all plastic or all metal cannulae should be employed (Fig. 52).

Dissection of tissue

Laparoscopic dissection is a combination of manipulation, retraction, sharp and blunt dissection, haemostasis, and suction and irrigation. The ideal dissection technique requires a modality which:

• Achieves dissection with haemostasis.
• Will be tissue selective and cause no inadvertent damage.
• Is safe for all: patient, surgeon and theatre staff.
• Is efficient in performance.
• The surgeon is familiar with its use and limitations.
• Is easily maintained and cost effective.

In practice, the majority of surgeons will continue to use combinations of different types of instruments and energy sources. However, instrument changes can be frustrating and time consuming but can be minimized by using each instrument for more than one purpose. For example, most non-traumatic, insulated, grasping forceps can be used for grasping, retracting, blunt dissection and coagulation. Insulated scissors can be used for sharp and blunt dissection as well as retraction of tissues by pushing and lifting

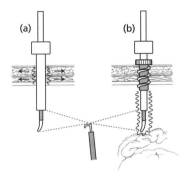

Fig. 52 An ideal situation for indirect coupling. (a) All metal cannulae allow dissipation of energy through the abdominal wall; (b) a plastic anchoring device prevents dissipation of energy, thereby causing sparks and burns at the cannula and instruments.

manoeuvres. An insulated suction irrigation probe may work as a suction and irrigation device, coagulator, blunt dissector and retractor. The harmonic scalpel can coagulate and divide tissue at the same time. Some disposable automatic clip applicators have means for dividing tissues in between clips. As a rule the tip of all instruments, particularly sharp ones, entering, moving or leaving the abdominal cavity must be kept under direct vision (Fig. 53).

Manipulation

As in open surgery, structures and tissue planes are exposed by gentle manipulation using atraumatic grasping forceps. The side (not tip) of any blunt instrument (scissors, grasping forceps, diathermy probe, suction probe), may be used to gently sweep, lift, or push tissues or structures. Exposure may be enhanced by gravity shifts (patient's position) and appropriate retraction (see page 55).

Sharp dissection

- Scissors: with or without diathermy.
- Diathermy probes: monopolar cutting, blended, or coagulating current through needle, fine hook, or edge of spatula diathermy probes are commonly used for sharp dissection. However, a bipolar cutting mode is being developed.
- Scalpel: rarely used in laparoscopy.
- Laser and ultrasound (see page 73, 76).

Blunt dissection

Once the appropriate tissue plane is opened by sharp dissection (scissors, diathermy), blunt dissection can be performed by the following means.

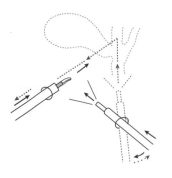

Fig. 53 The tip of all functioning instruments must be in view when entering the abdominal cavity, approaching and moving within the operating field, and leaving the abdominal cavity.

Instruments

Open and close the jaws of scissors or atraumatic grasping forceps (double jaw action instruments are preferred). The tip of all blunt instruments such as grasping forceps, or diathermy or suction/ irrigation probes may also be used.

Pledget swab dissection

Be aware of pledget dislodgement during both dissection and withdrawal, particularly through the flap valve cannulae.

Stripping

Using one or two atraumatic insulated grasping forceps, strands of connective tissues and fine adhesions can easily and effectively be separated from their attachments by gentle pulling. Exposed blood vessels are dealt with in the appropriate manner. However, the disadvantages of the technique are:
• Minor oozing of blood which can be dealt with by diathermy via the insulated grasping forceps.
• Shredding or perforation of viscera, if the attachments are strong. Here, the bands may be disrupted in between two forceps (Fig. 54).

Haemostasis

Bleeding during laparoscopic surgery, is the commonest cause of conversion to open surgery, particularly for those who are less experienced laparoscopic surgeons. Bleeding can be difficult to control because:
• Access may be limited.
• Unlike open surgery, in laparoscopy one is not always able to apply direct pressure.
• Cut vessels rapidly retract within surrounding tissues.
• Bleeding can obscure the view by:
  (a) Directly hitting the telescope.
  (b) Blood absorbs light and the view becomes poor especially with smaller telescopes.

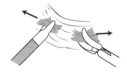

Fig. 54 Strands of connective tissues can safely be disrupted in between two forceps.

(c) Blood clots can be difficult to clear with 5 mm suction probes due to their small diameter.

Accordingly, prevention of haemorrhage must remain the most important principle in laparoscopic surgery. Before they are cut, small vessels should be diathermized with either bipolar or unipolar coagulation current, and large vessels should be clipped, ligated or stapled. However, the recently developed ultrasound activated scalpel or shears appear to have excellent coagulation and cutting properties, all in one, for vessels up to 2 mm in diameter (see page 76). A suction, irrigation system must always be ready to use, which allows the identification of bleeding points prior to their securement, washes away blood clots and tissue debris, and clears smoke.

It is well worth remembering that during laparoscopic viewing a minor bleeding point may appear major because of the magnifying effect of the telescope.

Suction/irrigation

A variety of dedicated suction/irrigation devices have been developed to replace a drip stand/saline bag and conventional suction unit. Irrigating saline is delivered under pressure of 100–500 mmHg by a pressurised CO_2 container. The device must have valves to prevent CO_2 being pumped into the abdominal cavity when the saline runs out. The use of heparin (1000 units/l) minimizes clot formation, large clots being difficult to aspirate. The suction/irrigation probe should have a single channel for both functions, with the flow controlled by a user friendly hand-held valve system of an appropriate size. Some probes are adapted to incorporate monopolar diathermy (Fig. 55).

Problems and solutions

• Two channel probes (half for suction, half for irrigation) provide inadequate suction mode and are best avoided.

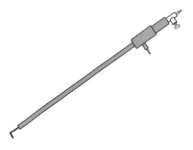

Fig. 55 Suction probe with a built-in monopolar diathermy probe.

- Bulky and difficult to operate valve systems can be frustrating and time consuming.
- Clogging of channel/valves by clots, loose tissue, debris and stones.
- Rapid loss of pneumoperitoneum with high and prolonged suction. Always try not to suck above the level of fluid (Fig. 56), but insert the tip of the suction device into the fluid 'sump'.
- High irrigation pressure may splash fluid onto the telescope and disturb the view.
- Omentum, appendices epiploicae, peritoneum, mesentery, or even bowel may get sucked into the suction probe and be very difficult to detach. When this happens, the system should be switched from suction mode into neutral or irrigation mode, and a pair of atraumatic graspers used through another working cannula to gently release the tissue.

Laser

Laser offers surgical cutting, coagulation and vaporization properties of high precision. However, electrocautery provides very adequate cutting and coagulation modalities for laparoscopic surgery. Surgical lasers, which are usable for minimal access surgery include: CO_2, argon, potassium titenyl phosphate (KTP) and neodymium-yttrium aluminium garnet (Nd-YAG) lasers. Their properties depend upon the characteristics of the laser beam, the nature and the colour of

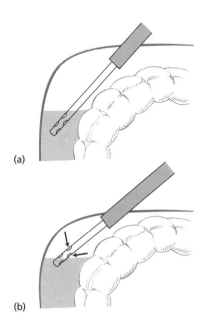

(a)

Fig. 56 Suction of peritoneal fluid. (a) Correct method; (b) incorrect suction above the level of fluid allows loss of pneumoperitoneum.

(b)

the structure in its path, the irradiation spot size, and the exposure time. In the hands of experienced surgeons, laser irradiation appears safe and effective. The dangers of the lasers are:
- Damages structures in its path.
- The laser beam can be reflected off shiny surfaces, therefore it has the potential for inadvertent damage, outside the operative field.
- It burns beyond the target tissue.
- Reflection through the optics can damage the surgeon's eyes.
- Inadvertent activation of the laser beam may cause harm at the point of contact to anybody in the operating theatre.
- Cooling of the contact tips with CO_2 gas is necessary which may carry the risk of gas embolism.
- Contact tips require regular replacement and are very expensive. The pointed tips are so sharp they can cause mechanical injuries to viscera.

These risks can be minimized by avoiding the use of bare fibre lasers (non-contact laser), but instead, focusing the beam with a probe (contact tip laser). Since the laser beam loses its power beyond the contact tip, burns beyond the target tissue and reflections are not a concern. Bleeding is the main indication for the use of non-contact laser, while cutting or excision are achievable by both bare fibres or contact tips. Another advantage of bare fibre non-contact beam is the large range of angles of delivery available during the procedure.

Contact probes (tips) can be made in various shapes such as ball tip for vaporization, flat for coagulation, and cones or blade for cutting (Fig. 57).

These tips are usually made from highly heat conducting sapphire or glass ceramics. Other advantages of contact tip lasers are:
- As the energy is focused, much lower laser power is necessary to produce the desired effect.
- The contact provides the surgeon with some tactile sensation.

CO_2 laser

The CO_2 creates an infrared invisible beam, which requires a second

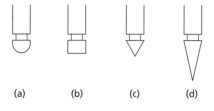

(a) (b) (c) (d)

Fig. 57 Contact laser applicators. (a) Ball tip for vaporization; (b) flat for coagulation; (c and d) cone and blade for cutting (sides may be used for coagulation).

low power red helium–neon laser as a guide beam. It is necessary for the beam to be delivered via air or gas media, therefore it cannot be used through optical fibres. The CO_2 laser is well absorbed by water-containing tissue to a depth of 0.2 mm with very little lateral propagation. These properties, make the CO_2 laser a precise vaporizing and cutting beam. The main disadvantages of the CO_2 laser are:

- A rigid articulated system with mirrors is required to deliver the beam.
- It produces smoke that can absorb energy and cause poor imaging. Therefore, a smoke extractor is required during laparoscopy.
- It gives poor coagulation properties.

Argon laser

This green–blue visible laser can be delivered through optical fibres and directed by both non-contact and contact modes. Its absorption is greatest by haemoglobin and melanin containing fluids and tissues, and has very little effect on clear fluids and tissues. Argon penetrates to 1 mm, and produces good coagulation, but not of large vessels. High power density can provide some vaporization and cutting properties.

KTP (potassium titenyl phosphate) laser

This lime green laser beam is primarily absorbed by haemoglobin and pigment containing tissues, and is not absorbed by clear fluids. The beam is conveyed by optical fibres and applied through both contact and non-contact mode. Tissue penetration of KTP is around 1 mm and therefore can be used for both coagulation and cutting purposes.

Nd–YAG (neodymium–yttrium aluminium garnet) laser

This 'near infrared' invisible laser requires an additional He–Ne guide beam. Nd–YAG laser passes through water with no effect and is absorbed by tissue proteins to a depth of 4 mm. It is a good coagulator and controls active haemorrhage well. This laser is transmittable through optical fibres. Its unfocused 'non-contact mode' beam can cause widespread injury to tissues; however, its contact mode is reliable. The Nd–YAG laser produces more lateral tissue propagation than the CO_2 laser.

High intensity focused ultrasound

Ultrasound is an acoustic longitudinal wave which consists of high and low pressure points which give it a mechanical energy. Ultrasound can propagate in solid, liquid and gas media at a frequency above 20 000 Hz (audible sound 20–20 000 cycles/s) without causing bulk motion of the media.

Ultrasound has been used for decades as an effective and non-invasive method of imaging tissues. The power used in diagnostic imaging is low and produces no measurable tissue effects. A higher output of power 'high intensity focused ultrasound' can provide therapeutic functions. Initially this was used for the fragmentation of stones in the urinary system, but subsequently has been developed for tissue dissection (fragmentation, coagulation, cutting) in both open and laparoscopic surgery.

There are two systems of high energy ultrasound which may be used for tissue dissection: ultrasound cavitational aspirator, and the ultrasound activated scalpel/shears.

Ultrasound cavitational aspirator

The system is composed of a generator which provides electrical energy, and a hand probe that houses the ultrasonic transducer. Its energy is delivered as a 23 000 Hz vibration with a longitudinal displacement of 300 μm. The hand piece, has a covering tube which provides irrigation and aspiration. The irrigant fluid dissipates thermal energy that generated from the mechanical energy of the acoustic waves, whilst the aspiration clears tissue debris for better tissue coupling.

The vibrations generate forces that fragment cells or expand tissue planes (cavitational mechanism). Low water content collagen rich tissues require much more energy to fragment than high water or fat content tissue such as liver and mesentery. This tissue selectivity allows a reliable dissection of tissues, such as liver and parenchymal tumour, with preservation of vessels, nerves and ductal structures.

Disadvantages

- Loss of pneumoperitoneum from aspiration. This effect may be minimized by higher laparoscopic insufflation gas flow.
- The irrigant fluid tends to disturb laparoscopic imaging by mist and splashing onto the telescope.
- An expensive tool with a limited use.

Ultrasound activated scalpel/shears (harmonic scalpel, laparoscopic coagulating shears)

A new ultrasonic coagulating and cutting system has been developed for use in laparoscopic surgery. It consists of a generator, and a hand piece which houses the ultrasonic transducer. Its ultrasonic energy is delivered as 55 000 Hz vibrations with a maximum longitudinal displacement of 80 μm by either a hook-blade (scalpel) or a shears (grasper). The basic mechanism for coagulating blood vessels by high energy ultrasound is similar to that of diathermy and laser. Vessels are sealed by pressure and coaption with a denatured protein coagulum. As the thermal energy generated by this system remains under 80 °C, necrosis and charring are minimal.

The hook blade produces an excellent balance of coagulation and cutting. Its sharp edge is used for cutting relatively avascular tissue. However, its flat side can be used as a coagulator (vessels less than 2 mm in diameter) if left vibrating for a few seconds (Fig. 58).

The shears have one blade which moves and the other is fixed. The moveable blade is called the clamp pad and holds unsupported tissue (peritoneum, mesentery, pedicles) within the shears against the fixed blade, which then delivers the energy (Fig. 59). The fixed blade has two edges, one of which is sharp and can be used for cutting relatively avascular tissue. The other edge is blunt and can be used for coagulating and then cutting tissue containing blood vessels upto 2 mm in diameter (experimental 5 mm vessel). The fixed blade can be rotated within the device to select the required edge at any given time.

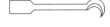

Fig. 58 Ultrasonic hook-blade (scalpel) applicator.

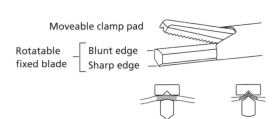

Moveable clamp pad

Rotatable fixed blade — Blunt edge / Sharp edge

Fig. 59 Ultrasonic shears.

Coagulating   Cutting

77

Advantages

- An efficient and easy system to use for coagulation and cutting tissues.
- It produces slight mist, but no smoke.
- No risk of electrical injury.

Disadvantages

- Lateral damage can occur, and cavitation at tissue planes may cause serious damage, albeit very rarely.
- Unlike the cavitational aspirator, the scalpel/shears are non-tissue selective.
- Expensive.

High velocity water jet

The system consists of a hydrodynamic device which produces kinetic energy through a fine pressurized water jet. It was introduced for conventional hepatic dissection, and is not yet suitable for endoscopic use without major modifications.

Hydrodissector

This device separates tissue planes and breaks down fat globules by pulsatile irrigation with crystalloid solution. The system has been used sporadically for laparoscopic procedures such as pelvic lymphadenectomy.

Ligation and suturing

Needle holder

Laparoscopic needle holders are similar in design to those used for conventional surgery (Fig. 60).

Requirements for laparoscopic needle holders:
- Grip the needle securely, preventing needle slide and swivel.
- Grip the needle at different angles.
- Allow easy internal knotting (curved needle holder may be better than straight).
- Handles which sit and easily rotate in surgeon's hand may be better than conventional angled handles (Fig. 60a).
- Reflection free, easily cleaned and sterilizable.

Although a spring operated needle holder grasps the needle in a fixed angle which does not slide and swivel, it is too traumatic to the suture material which makes internal knotting difficult (Fig. 60d).

Some of these needle holders grasp the needle at a particular angle and therefore more than one needle holder will be required during any one procedure.

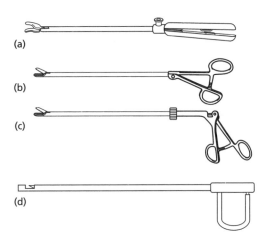

(a)

(b)

(c)

(d)

Fig. 60 Needle holders. (a) Straight handle; (b and c) scissors type straight and angled handle; (d) spring operated.

Needles/sutures

Although ski needles, with a round or triangular body, and straight needles are made specifically for endoscopic use, conventional curved needles are used more commonly. The inner calibre of the cannula limits the use of large curved needles.

Knotting

Proper knotting is essential to secure vessels, ligate ductal structures and perform anastomoses.

External knotting

External slip knot. The Roeder knot, is the most reliable external one way slip knot (Fig. 61) which works best with dry catgut and to a lesser degree with silk. The security of this knot improves with hydration by tissue fluid. This knot is slightly less safe with material such as PDS, Vicryl, proline or nylon caused by the low friction coefficient which allows two way slipping. However, double throws at the beginning and end should add additional security (Fig. 62).

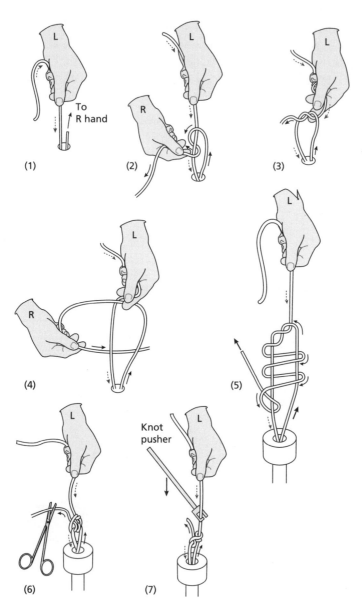

Fig. 61 Extracorporeal Roeder knot, steps 1–7. Arrows indicate direction of suture movement/placement (broken arrow, fixed limb/out–in part of suture; solid arrow, knotting manoeuvre/in–out).

External surgeon's knot. A familiar knot to all surgeons who work with all suture materials (Fig. 63). However, materials such as catgut and silk do not slide easily.

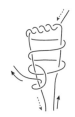

Fig. 62 Modification of Roeder knot
(double throws at beginning and end).

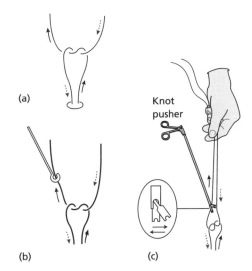

(a)

Knot
pusher

Fig. 63 Extracorporeal surgeon's knot.
(a) Surgeon's knot; (b and c) tying the
first throw with two different types of
knot pushers.

(b)   (c)

Internal knotting

The most widely practised knotting in laparoscopic surgery is internal knotting. Initially, it is difficult to learn, is time consuming and often frustrating. However, with practice, it can be performed safely, securely, smoothly and quickly. The number and type of locking throws are determined by the type of suture material used, and site and the purpose for which the suture will be applied (Fig. 64).

• One needle holder and one grasper (as a receptive instrument) are required.

• A curved receptive grasper may facilitate knotting.

• Two needle holders allow two way stitching to and fro.

• For interrupted suturing or ligating, a short suture (10–15 cm) is easier to knot. With experience, however, long sutures may be used.

• The tail should be kept short, and the long limb is placed near the end of the suture.

• A needle may or may not be attached to the suture used.

• An attached needle makes knotting easier when held near its tip in the line of the receptive instrument (interrupted suture only).

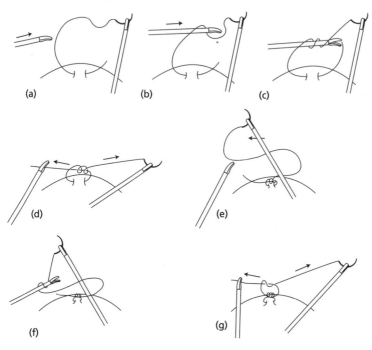

Fig. 64 Intracorporeal knotting. Arrows indicate direction of movement. (a) Keep a short tail and the long limb is placed near the end with the needle held near its tip in the line of the receptive instrument; (b,c,d) stages of tying the first double throw; (e,f,g) the second throw is completed in reverse order.

• The suture material may be damaged and weakened by rough handling. A rubber shod grasper minimizes damage but can make knotting more tedious.
• If the needle is still attached, the suture is introduced into the peritoneal cavity (Fig. 65):

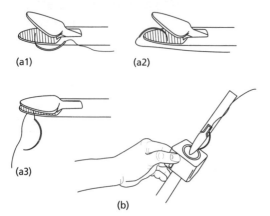

Fig. 65 (a,1–3) Methods of holding needle/suture; (b) introduction of suture/needle into the peritoneal cavity.

(a) by inserting the curved needle with its point in the tip of the needle holder jaws and its long axis along that of the needle holder. A safe technique, but requires a larger than usual cannula (10 mm cannula for 3/o suture) (Fig. 65a1).

(b) or by placing the needle with its point deep in the jaws (Fig. 65a2). Using this technique, 4/o suture curved needles, slightly straightened out larger curved needles, ski and straight needles can be introduced into the peritoneal cavity through 5 mm cannulae. To prevent visceral injury, however, it is absolutely critical that the tip of the instrument (end of the needle) is kept under direct vision at the time of introduction.

(c) or by grasping the suture near the needle (Fig. 65a3). This may weaken or damage the suture, hence it is not a good technique for continuous suturing. Also needles, particularly curved needles, may jam inside the cannula and therefore a larger than usual cannula may be needed.

• For the first throw, a single loop for catgut, and a double loop for other sutures may be necessary.

• To avoid visceral injury, the tip of an attached needle must always be kept under direct vision. Alternatively, the needle is detached and removed prior to knotting.

• A needle holder or grasper with a jaw opening mechanism that lies flush with the shaft of the instrument greatly facilitates knotting by allowing the loops of suture to easily slide off the shaft of the instrument without being caught in the instrument (Fig. 66).

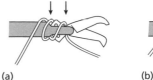

Fig. 66 Instrument designs that might affect suturing technique. (a) suture caught in the instrument; (b) suture slides off the instrument.

(a)   (b)

Ligatures

Pretied ligature

A commercially available pretied (Roeder slip knot) loop of suture material threaded through a push rod with or without suture introducer (Fig. 67). This item is suitable for:

• Ligation of ductal structures such as the appendix, or divided cystic duct or ureter.

• Securing an already diathermized/clipped and divided pedicle or vessels.

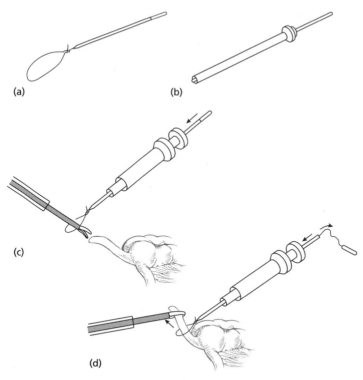

Fig. 67 Pretied knot/suture ligature. (a) A pretied suture with its push rod; (b) the device within the applicator; (c) grasping instrument placed through the loop; (d) the tissue pulled through the loop which is then tightened securely.

- Closure of a small perforation of the gall bladder.
- Closure of a small peritoneal gap.

Ligature using an extracorporeal knot

To ligate with the external knot before the structure is divided (Fig. 68). Figure 61 (page 80) demonstrates the technique of extracorporeal knotting. The main disadvantage of this technique is damage of the tissue by serration from the suture during the withdrawal process and knot sliding. The damaging effect may be lessened by a grasper/ needle holder inserted inside the loop to take the tension off the structure (Fig. 68c,d).

Ligature using an intracorporeal knot

To avoid damage to the tissue by serration, a piece of suture material,

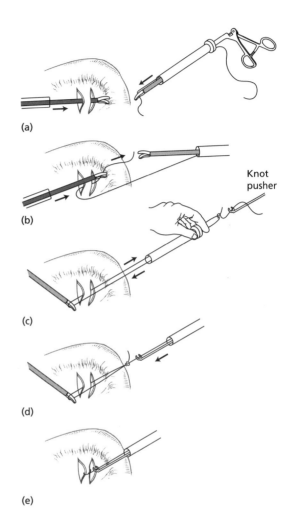

Fig. 68 Ligature using an extracorporeal knot. (a) An appropriate length of suture introduced into the peritoneal cavity; (b) the end of suture fed around the tissue to be ligated by a second grasper; (c) the end of suture pulled out through the cannula for external knotting. To prevent gas leak a finger is kept on the cannula. A curved/angled grasping forceps inside the loop prevents serration of the tissue; (d,e) a knot pusher completes the ligature.

with or without a needle attached, may be used to ligate before or after a vascular pedicle or ductal structure are divided (Fig. 69).

Suturing

Laparoscopic suturing requires considerable training and practice. The basic principle of suturing is similar to that of open surgery. Any atraumatic suture material on a straight, ski shaped or curved needle may be used. However, the shape and size of the needle depends on the size of the cannula used. The access cannulae are placed, preferably in front, and on one or both sides of the telescope with the two suturing instruments meeting in front of the telescope at

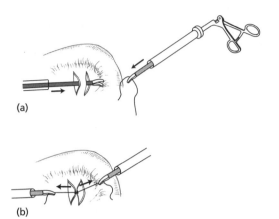

(a)

(b)

Fig. 69 Ligature using an intracorporeal knot. (a) A short piece of suture introduced and placed around the tissue to be ligated; (b) the suture is tied using internal knotting.

about a 45–125° angle (optimal 65°) (see page 49, Fig. 30). The technique of suturing requires a needle holder to introduce and drive the needle; another needle holder or a grasper (receptive instrument) to manipulate and align the tissue, to receive and pull the needle, and to assist in knotting. During continuous suturing, a rubber shod grasper through a third, but convenient, access cannula is recommended to hold tension on the suture and stabilize the suture line (Fig. 70).

• Large ports (10 mm) extend the surgeons options during suturing especially the size of needles that can be used.

• Prepare and align the tissue for suturing.

• Laparoscopic tissue clamps may be required to stabilize tissues and prevent bleeding and leakage from hollow organs as in gastro-intestinal anastomosis.

• The suture is introduced into the abdominal cavity by grasping either the needle or the suture (Fig. 65).

• Two needle holders allow two way needle drive to and fro.

• An ordinary curved needle is the most suitable needle to use for both interrupted and continuous suturing.

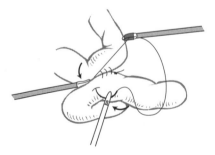

Fig. 70 Continuous internal suturing. Needle-holder drives the needle; second needle holder/grasping forceps aligns and stabilizes the suture line, and receives the needle; rubber-shod grasper keeps tension on the suture and stabilizes the suture line.

- The initial terminal fixation of any suture line may be achieved by either a standard internal reef knot (most widely used), a pretied slip knot loop or a metal clip. The latter may be unreliable because the clip may slip off.
- To avoid damaging internal organs in between bites, hold the tip of the needle towards the abdominal wall.
- The end terminal fixation of the suture line is achieved by an internal reef knot, Edinburgh slip knot, or even a metal clip (clip may be unreliable).
- The length of the suture requires careful judgement because tangling may be a problem particularly with materials such as PDS, maxon, proline and nylon sutures.

Ligature clips

Ligature clips are made of metal or absorbable plastic (Fig. 71). The metal clips are either stainless steel or titanium. They are available in lengths of 6, 9 and 11 mm. The stainless steel clip has the highest mechanical performance and is well tolerated by body tissues but produces significant local artefacts on computerized tomography (CT) and magnetic resonance imaging (MRI). Titanium clips perform well mechanically, are inert to tissues, and produce very little local artefacts on imaging. The absorbable clips perform reasonably well (have a delicate locking system) and are radiotransparent.

Metal clip appliers are either reusable, single or automatic multiload 10 mm instruments with or without a rotatable shaft, or disposable automatic multiload 10 or 5 mm instruments with a rotatable shaft. Absorbable clips whether single or multiload, require a specific 10 mm instrument which is reusable.

The reusable single load appliers are inexpensive instruments, but require re-loading outside the abdomen after each clip application. They work well when a few clips are needed as in cholecystectomy,

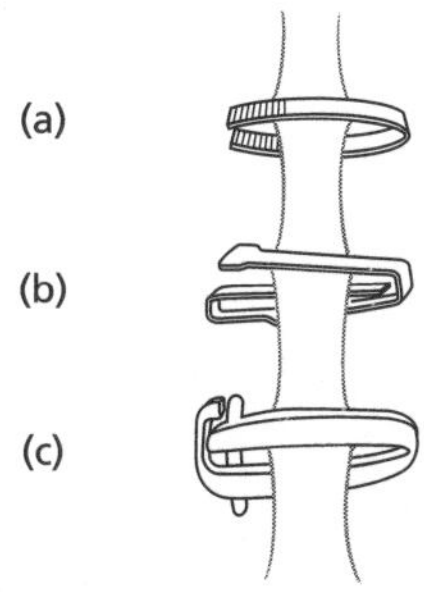

(a)

(b)

(c)

Fig. 71 Ligature clips. (a) Metal single loop; (b) metal double loop; (c) absorbable plastic.

87

biopsy, appendicectomy or testicular vessel ligation. The disposable and multiload reusable instruments, on the other hand, are capable of firing up to 15–30 clips (eight for reusable instruments) in rapid succession. They are expensive instruments, but can greatly facilitate procedures in which multiple ligatures are needed as in bowel resection or splenectomy. Some disposable models have hooks and blades built into the shaft for isolating and dividing structures all at one application.

Ligature clips may be used to:
• Ligate vessels.
• Close luminal structures such as cystic duct, ureter, or even appendix stump. ,
• Fix terminal ends of sutures.
• Mark site of organs such as stomach following fundoplication and ovary after ovariopexy for pelvic radiation.

1 The structure to be divided is dissected circumferentially for a length allowing the application of one to three clips on the patient's side and one clip distally.
2 The clip applier should approach the structure to be ligated at an angle that allows the surgeon to view the jaws of the instrument side on (Figs 53 and 72).

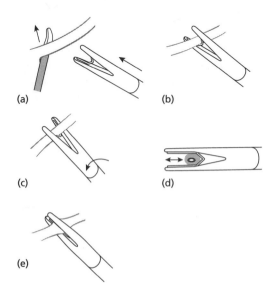

(a)

(b)

(c)

(d)

(e)

Fig. 72 Steps of applying a clip. (a) The applier should approach the target at full view; (b,c) the applier is positioned across the structure making sure that no other tissues are caught within the jaws by rotating the applier sideways and seeing the lower jaw clear of the surrounding tissues before the clip is closed; (d,e) the clip must pass across the structure to be ligated before it is closed.

3 With the single load 'reusable' instrument, the clip may dislodge from the applier while approaching the target.

4 To ensure safe occlusion, the clip must pass across the structure (Fig. 72d,e).

5 After placing the first clip, the closed applier may be used to stabilize and gently tent the tissue while the second 'grasping' instrument is replaced (Fig. 73).

6 If necessary suture ligature with internal knotting or an endo loop, applied proximally, should provide additional security to the divided structure (Fig. 74).

Stapling or tacking clips

These metal clips close in either a rectangular configuration as do skin closure staples, or 'B' configuration. Corkscrew clips that keep appliances in place with their twisted shape, are also available. The appliers are usually disposable automatic multiload 11 mm instruments with a rotatable shaft (5 mm instrument for corkscrew clips). Some models have a flexible end to help align the instrument with the structures (Fig. 75).

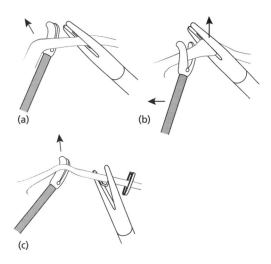

(a)　　　　　(b)

(c)

Fig. 73 Steps of applying a second clip. (a) After placing the first clip; (b) the structure, still held by the closed stapler, is lifted gently while the grasper is repositioned further along the structure; (c) the closed grasper is gently lifted while the applier is repositioned to deliver the second clip.

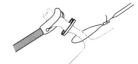

Fig. 74 A proximal suture ligature provides additional security.

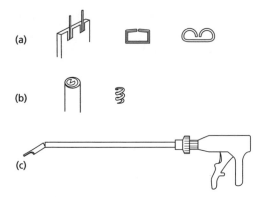

Fig. 75 Stapling clips. (a) Rectangular or B-configuration clips; (b) corkscrew clips; (c) automatic multiload applier with a rotatable and flexible end.

Stapling/tacking clips may be used to:
- To fix patches of mesh to abdominal wall defects such as inguinal herniae and diaphragmatic herniae.
- To close peritoneal incisions.
- As an alternative to interrupted sutures.

One or two grasping forceps are required to prepare and approximate the edges of the tissues/mesh before placing a clip.

After placing the first clip, the two approximated edges still held by the applier, are kept under gentle tension while the grasping forceps are moved to approximate edges further along the line (Fig. 76).

Linear staplers

The linear stapler device with a rotatable shaft is a disposable

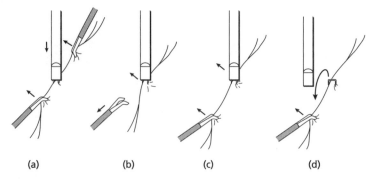

Fig. 76 Steps of internal stapling. (a) The edges are approximated and stabilized by two grasping forceps while placing the first staple; (b,c) the edges still held by the closed stapler are kept under tension while the front grasper is repositioned further away from the first staple; (d) the edges still held by the front closed grasper are kept under tension while the stapler is moved along the line to apply the second staple (e).

instrument which can be loaded up to four times (Fig. 77). The cartridge loading units come in lengths of 30 mm and 60 mm, each delivering four to six separate rows of metal staples with a knife to cut the tissue in the middle. The staple sizes are 2.5 mm (vascular) or 3.5–4.8 mm (regular). The longer staples are used for bowel, vagina and bladder.

• The size 30 device requires a 12 mm cannula, and the size 60 device requires 15 or 18 mm cannula.

• A special gauge instrument is available to measure the thickness of the tissue to be occluded.

• It is important to ensure that the staple lines pass across the structure to be occluded. If this is not possible, a second cartridge can be used.

Sewing device

Suturing and knotting in laparoscopic surgery require considerable practice and are time consuming. In an attempt to facilitate suturing, various sewing devices in both disposable and reusable forms, have been developed (Fig. 78). However, they have not gained popularity yet because:

• They are expensive.
• Still requiring some practice.
• They have a very limited choice of suture material, length of needle and length of suture.
• They require space to manoeuvre.

Tissue glue/sealant

Recently, there have been several reports describing haemostasis and closure of gastrointestinal defects by the use of the laparoscopic

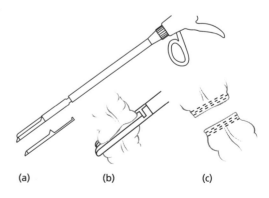

Fig. 77 Linear stapler. (a) Multifire rotatable linear stapler with a spare cartridge; (b) the stapler across the colon; (c) divided colon with three separate rows of metal clips on each side occluding the colon.

(a)   (b)   (c)

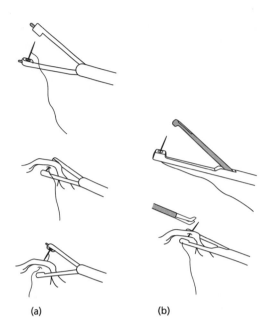

(a)　　　　　　(b)

Fig. 78 Sewing devices. (a) Disposable; (b) reusable.

application of tissue fibrin glue. The sealant initially plugs the hole. Definitive closure occurs as a result of an inflammatory process ultimately leading to epithelialization. So far, experience is limited to experimental work, and clinical case reports of haemostasis in minor or venous bleeds, and sealing of peptic ulcer perforations, biliary leakage, minor traumatic rupture of the spleen and liver, fistulas and intestinal anastomosis.

Specimen extraction

Tissue specimens, stones and foreign bodies may be extracted from the abdominal cavity via the cannula, an enlarged cannula site, or a selectively placed minilaparotomy incision. The choice largely depends on the nature and the size of the specimens, and to a lesser degree cosmesis. A retrieval bag, with or without tissue fragmentation may prove necessary in some cases.

Extraction direct through the cannula

This method is suitable for specimens which are small enough to pass through the laparoscopic cannulae. Examples are:
- Biopsy specimens
- Stones (spilled out of gall bladder, bile duct, kidney and ureter)

- Foreign bodies
- Collapsible structure such as the non-inflamed gall bladder and cysts (ovarian, mesenteric, renal)
- Appendix.

However, specimens may impact in the cannula (usually at the level of the valve), or fall back into the peritoneal cavity where it may be difficult to find amongst loops of bowels. The manoeuvre must therefore be kept under laparoscopic view at all times (Fig. 79). Occasionally, the telescope (same size or smaller) may have to be changed to another cannula in which case the operative view, and hand–eye co-ordination may become more difficult.

Extraction through the cannula site

Large tissue specimens can be extracted via a cannula site. While the site of the umbilical cannula provides a cosmetically superior scar, it may not be the easiest route and has a higher risk of port site herniation. Additionally, it requires a change of telescope which may lead to a less adequate laparoscopic view and difficulty with hand–eye co-ordination. When there is a risk of contamination (infective,

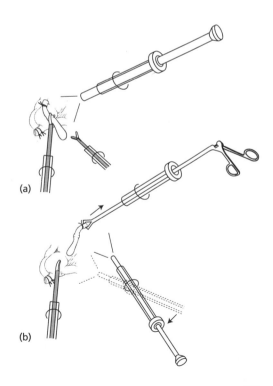

Fig. 79 Extraction of specimen (appendix) through a cannula. (a) Appendicectomy and preparation of the appendix for extraction using a 10 mm telescope through the primary cannula; (b) a 5 mm telescope is placed through the left lower secondary cannula while a toothed grasping forceps is used through the primary cannula to extract the appendix.

malignant), or a need for fragmentation of tissue, a retrieval bag may be necessary.

Technique without a bag

This technique is suitable for benign, non-friable cystic specimens (gall bladder, ovarian cyst, cystic or dilated kidney), or foreign bodies.

The specimen is prepared for removal. Large cysts or dilated kidneys may be aspirated before extraction. A large-toothed grasping forceps is passed through the selected cannula (the larger the cannula the better). The specimen is then grasped (gall bladder in the region of neck) and gently manoeuvred into the cannula, and both the specimen and the cannula are now extracted from the abdomen through the cannula site (Fig. 80a,b). This will be followed by a sudden loss of pneumoperitoneum. To continue with further laparoscopy, the cannula site has to be plugged with a finger, re-insertion of a cannula, or suturing of the wound.

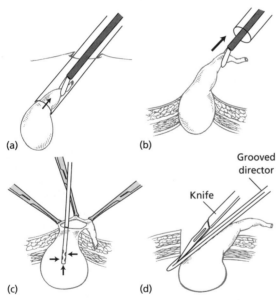

(a)   (b)

(c)   (d)

Grooved director

Knife

Fig. 80 Extraction of specimen (gall bladder) through the cannula site without a retrieval bag. (a,b) The specimen is grasped, gently manoeuvred into the cannula, and both the specimen and the cannula are extracted from the abdomen; (c) a large specimen may be opened externally and its contents aspirated/removed before the specimen is extracted; (d) the wound may be enlarged with a grooved director to protect the specimen and a knife.

If the specimen is too large to deliver (Fig. 8oc,d), the specimen is opened externally and its contents are aspirated with the sucker. Stones may be crushed and removed using appropriate forceps. If necessary, the wound may be enlarged and must be closed completely after the procedure, using a J needle.

Problems and solutions

• Infected or malignant specimens cause contamination and thereby increase the risks of wound infection, postoperative wound disruption and hernia, and malignant cell implantation. Here, a retrieval bag should be used.

• During extraction excess force may cause tissue disruption, spillage of contents (stones) and contamination (Fig. 81).

• A change of telescope from one cannula to another may be required to allow easier extraction. This may lead to inadequate laparoscopic viewing and difficult hand and eye co-ordination (Fig. 30, page 49).

• This technique is difficult in obese patients.

Retrieval bag

While a simple plastic bag or a condom may be effective for removal

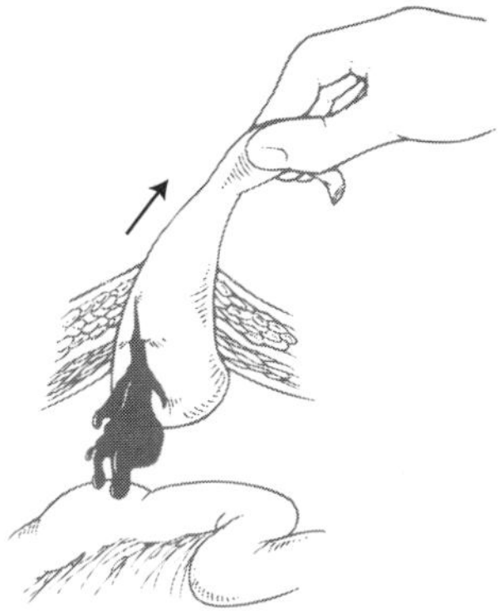

Fig. 81 During extraction of specimen excess force may cause tissue disruption, spillage of contents and contamination.

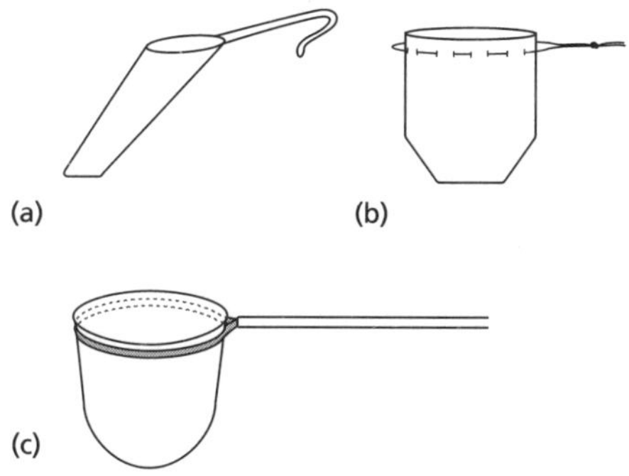

(a)   (b)

Fig. 82 Different types of retrieval bags. (a) With a built-in tail for manoeuvre; (b) with a purse-string; (c) with a built-in, spring metal band and introducer.

(c)

95

of some specimens, they carry the risk of rupture and spillage of contents which cause contamination and markedly prolong the procedure. Purpose designed laparoscopic bags come in various sizes and forms (Fig. 82) with or without built-in introducers and purse-strings. A bag for entrapment and extraction of specimens should be strong, easily manoeuvrable, and impermeable to microorganisms and tissue cells.

Technique with a bag

A bag is required to trap and extract specimens such as:
- Malignant tissue to avoid seeding.
- An infected gall bladder containing stones to avoid peritoneal contamination and spillage of stones which can be difficult to retrieve.
- A large infected appendix to avoid peritoneal contamination.
- Small segments of bowel (malignant/infective contamination).
- A kidney which may be large and require fragmentation before extraction (also malignant and infective contamination).
- A spleen which requires fragmentation and to avoid spillage of splenic tissue.

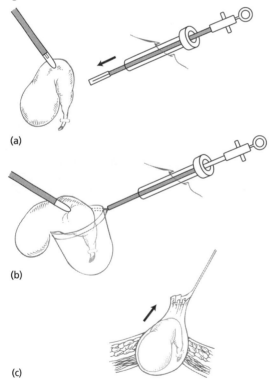

(a)

(b)

(c)

Fig. 83 Extraction of specimen (gall bladder) with a bag on its purpose-built introducer. (a) The device is introduced into the abdominal cavity; (b) the prepared specimen is placed inside the bag; (c) the bag containing the specimen is removed.

- Uterus and ovaries (fragmentation/malignant contamination).

A retrieval bag is introduced into the abdominal cavity through a large cannula, either on its purpose-built introducer (Fig. 83), or by using a grasping forceps with a reducing sleeve/diaphragm (Fig. 84).

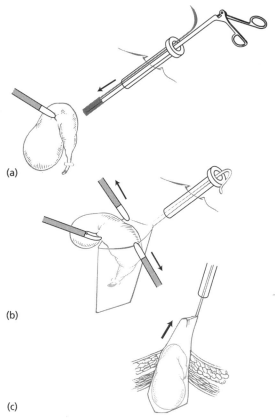

(a)

(b)

(c)

Fig. 84 Extraction of specimen (gall bladder) with a loose bag. (a) The bag is introduced into the abdominal cavity using a grasping forceps; (b) the bag is held open by two or three grasping forceps and the specimen is placed inside the bag; (c) the tail/purse-string is drawn out through the cannula and then the cannula and bag extracted.

A loose bag, may have to be placed completely within the abdomen, before its neck is opened. The specimen is then placed within the bag. The tail/string attached to the bag or the introducer is then drawn out of the cannula and the cannula and the bag extracted (Figs 83 and 84).

If the specimen is too large to deliver, the bag is opened externally and its contents are aspirated after fragmentation if necessary and then removed (Fig. 85a).

Tissue fragmentation may be achieved by a pair of grasping forceps or a purpose made morcellator. This procedure, has to be monitored laparoscopically as there is a risk of the bag being damaged. If necessary, the wound may be enlarged (Fig. 85b).

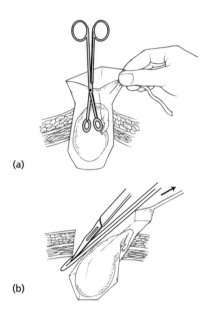

(a)

(b)

Fig. 85 Extraction of a large specimen from the abdominal cavity. (a) Contents of the bag aspirated/fragmented/morcellated/removed; (b) wound may be enlarged using a grooved director to protect the bag.

Problems and solutions. Placing the specimen in a bag can be a difficult manoeuvre. However, a purpose-made all in one bag, introducer, and a spring metal band that automatically opens and closes the bag diminishes the problem.

Damage to the plastic bag and condom can easily be made by excess traction and/or morcellation. A strong, purpose-made bag minimizes this risk particularly when morcellation is required.

Minilaparotomy for tissue removal

When the specimen is too large to deliver intact through an enlarged cannula site, an appropriately placed minilaparotomy incision allows the specimen to be removed from the abdomen. This technique is usually indicated in extensive laparoscopic intestinal surgery as in subtotal or hemicolectomy (colitis or carcinoma of colon). In difficult circumstances, a minilaparotomy incision may allow part of the procedure such as vascular or mesenteric division to be completed through the laparotomy incision, following laparoscopic mobilization of the organ in question.

Section 3
Setting up in the operating theatre

While purpose designed laparoscopic theatres may become available in the future, currently the performance of laparoscopic surgery has to be integrated into existing structures.

Hand instruments

Most instruments are expensive, delicate, and/or relatively complex in their construction, therefore care must be taken during handling, cleaning, sterilization and storage. Instruments that are used frequently may be packed together, while those which are used infrequently may be packed individually for use as needed. This exercise prolongs the life of the instruments, and lessens the need for unnecessary re-sterilization procedures. The surgeon and nursing assistant must be familiar with the ways in which instruments are prepared, stored and function.

Equipment

Although laparoscopy can be performed with one monitor, two are preferable so that the surgeon and assistant on either side of the operating table can see along a direct line.

The laparoscopic equipment is best placed on purpose designed trolleys with the monitors mounted at heights which are comfortable for the surgeon and the assistants.

The interconnection between various parts of the imaging equipment must be kept simple, easily workable and once set, left undisturbed by untrained individuals. For beginners, colour coding of interconnection wires in relation to input and output terminals can be very helpful.

The diathermy machine and laser apparatus are usually independently placed around the theatre.

Check list

Before any laparoscopic procedure is initiated, make sure that all of the required instruments and equipment are available and are functioning properly. The availability of spare instruments and equipment and supporting technicians are essential. The patient should never arrive in the operating theatre without being informed that the procedure may be converted to an open procedure when and if necessary.

Patient position and preparation

A nasogastric tube to empty the stomach is essential for safe placement of the Veress needle/cannulae in the upper abdomen or umbilical site. An empty bladder is essential during lower abdominal access and/or procedure. However, urinary catheterization is not always necessary, for example when the bladder is empty (thin adults and paediatric patients) and the procedure is short.

For laparoscopic surgery, most patients are placed in the supine position. Depending on the nature of the laparoscopic procedure and surgeon's preference (Fig. 86) the operator, assistant and scrubbed nurse may stand on either side of the table. In upper abdominal surgery, the operator may find a more comfortable position by standing between the patient's abducted legs (with or without hip and knee flexion). A modified Lloyd-Davies position (lithotomy position) is needed when performing a combined abdomino-perineal procedure or when operating on the oesophagus or stomach. In renal and suprarenal surgery a complete or partial lateral position is usually needed. Small children and infants may be positioned supine at the foot of the table. A degree of Trendelenburg, reverse-Trendelenburg, and/or lateral tilt may allow better access and exposure. When using the image intensifier, during bilateral procedures, or splenectomy alteration in the position of the operating table may be needed.

The skin is prepared from nipples to below the groin. The towels are placed so that the entire anterior abdominal wall is available for access at all times. Adhesive towels or tapes prevent instruments and cables falling between the towels and the patient. Transparent adhesive film (Opsite) to cover the whole abdomen should not be used as pieces of plastic may be pushed into the wounds by the trocar/cannula. A side pouch drape keeps some instruments and connections out of site but accessible.

An instrument holder or fixed retractor may be fixed to the operating table at this stage.

Setting up for the procedure

The height and angle of the first video screen should be adjusted to allow an ideal and comfortable working posture for the surgeon (usually at or just below the eye level at or near 90° to the line of surgeon and operative field).

The height and angle of second video screen (if available) should be adjusted for the assistant/scrub nurse. This screen may be placed on the same side as the first screen, the end of the table or more

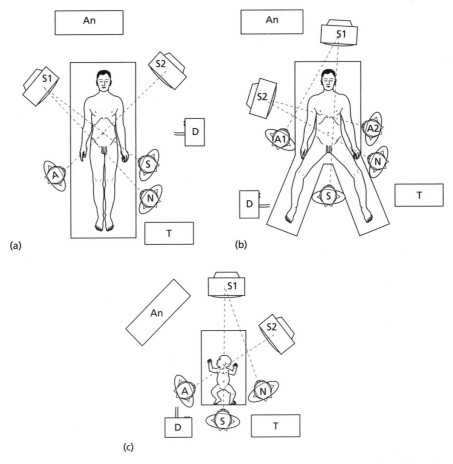

Fig. 86 Examples of theatre layout for upper abdominal surgery (a,b) adult and older children; (c) small children. S, Surgeon; A/A1/A2, assistants; N, nurse; S1/S2 screens; T, instrument trolley; D, diathermy/US/laser; An, anaesthetic apparatus.

often on the opposite side (depending on the nature of the procedure).

The insufflator should be visible to both the surgeon and the anaesthetist.

All the equipment must be accessible to the theatre technician for connection, adjustment and function.

The leads (cables, wires, tubes) are connected, placed and fixed to the towels in such a way that they cause the least obstruction to the operating team and prevent tangling. Care must be taken not to allow the non-sterile part of connections into the sterile operative field.

To minimize interference on the video screen during diathermy, plug the diathermy machine into a terminal separate to that of the video trolley and keep the diathermy lead separate from the camera lead.

Once a pneumoperitoneum is established and the primary cannula is in place, the telescope (keep the telescope in a warmer prior to use) is connected to both the camera and light source. Only then should the light source be switched on, as high intensity light can burn the patient and drape. Make sure that the interfaces between the telescope, camera and light cable are dry before connection, because moisture may distort imaging. Focus the camera and white balance (if required) before placing the telescope into the cannula. Further white balancing may be required at any subsequent telescope changes.

Section 4
Laparoscopic procedures

Diagnostic laparoscopy

There is no doubt about the values of diagnostic laparoscopy in all surgical specialities. The technique is simple and safe. However, its benefits are often enhanced if the surgeon is prepared and experienced with therapeutic laparoscopy. The ability to insert secondary cannulae, manipulate tissue, use diathermy and suction/irrigation, and perform laparoscopic haemostasis, adhesiolysis and biopsy are important before the diagnostic laparoscopy becomes an integral part of the surgeon's routine practice. The definitive therapeutic laparoscopic or open surgical procedure may be undertaken during the same anaesthetic if and when the circumstances are right.

Diagnostic laparoscopy may allow:
- Visualizing whether there is a problem or not.
- Localizing the pathology.
- Assessing the extent and the nature of the pathology (malignant, vascular, cystic) through vision, palpation with instruments and ultrasound probes.
- Knowing whether there is associated pathology such as metastases in malignant cases or portal hypertension in liver disease.
- Sampling fluid or tissue (aspiration, brush, washing, fine/trucut needle biopsy, punch or excision biopsy).
- Radiological imaging (cholangiography, angiography).

Indications

Acute

- Abdominal pain (diagnosis and fluid sampling) as in suspected appendicitis, tubo-ovarian pathology, diverticulitis, ischaemic bowel, perforation and obstruction.
- Trauma (diagnosis, assessment of severity and whether requires a definitive procedure) as in blunt injury, stab wound and air rifle injury.
- It is contraindicated in seriously ill or unstable patients, gunshot injury and high velocity missile injury.

Elective

- Hepatobiliary disease (assessment, cholangiography, angiography, staging, biopsy) as in biliary atresia, cirrhosis, hepatitis, primary or secondary liver lesions, benign neoplasia, cyst or vascular lesions and portal hypertension.

- Malignant conditions (operable or inoperable lesions, peritoneal deposits, lymph node or distant metastases, staging biopsy) as in oesophageal, gastric, intestinal or pancreatic cancer, Hodgkin's disease, gynaecological, prostatic or bladder cancer.
- Ascites (assessment, associated lesions, cytology) as in malignant or inflammatory disease, or cirrhosis of liver.
- Recurrent or chronic abdominal pain as in inflammatory appendix, pelvic or intestinal conditions, adhesions, Meckel's diverticulum.
- Impalpable testes (present or absent).
- Intersex (assessment, biopsy).

Instruments

While diagnostic laparoscopy may be achievable by using a single telescopic cannula with or without one or two secondary cannulae, one or two atraumatic grasping forceps, aspiration needle or biopsy forceps may be required. It is important that full laparoscopy and laparotomy sets are available for use at an immediate notice.

An operating telescope, incorporating both a telescope and a working channel, may prove useful in situations where diagnosis can be combined with a simple therapeutic measure. The examples are: assessment and sampling in suspected cancer; aspiration of ovarian cyst; removal of foreign body; and even laparoscopic assisted appendicectomy.

Technique

The patient is placed in the supine position. However, a lithotomy position may be necessary for pelvic organ assessment. A peri-umbilical primary (telescope) cannula serves most diagnostic procedures adequately. However, this position should be modified in the presence of a scar or other known lesions (see section on Access, pages 22, 30). The telescope is inserted and, if required, one or two secondary cannulae are then placed in either the upper abdomen (for upper abdominal conditions) or lower abdomen (for lower abdominal conditions). The exact number, site and size of the secondary cannulae depends on the patient's size and nature of the diagnostic procedure (Fig. 87).

As for conventional laparotomy, general inspection of the peritoneal cavity is followed by specific inspection of the suspected area of pathology. Exposure may be improved by head-up tilt for upper abdominal procedures, Trendelenburg for lower abdominal, and lateral tilts for lateral abdominal inspections.

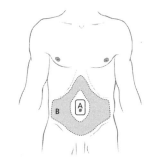

Fig. 87 Position of cannulae for diagnostic laparoscopy. A, Primary 'telescope' cannula; B, secondary 'working' cannulae — exact sites depend on the nature of the procedure.

An angled telescope (30/45°) may also facilitate the view. Liver, gall bladder, gastrointestinal tract, pelvic organs may require manipulation using palpating probes, atraumatic grasping forceps, retractors, or an ultrasound probe. The entire length of the small bowel may be inspected from ileocaecal valve to duodenojejunal flexure using two pairs of atraumatic grasping forceps (Fig. 88). Very steep Trendelenburg or lateral tilts may be required to assist para-aortic or iliac node inspection and biopsy. The pancreas may be exposed through a window in an avascular area of the gastrocolic omentum and by lifting the stomach and left lobe of the liver up. Pancreatic needle biopsy can be performed either directly or through the gastric wall.

Transhepatic cholangiography is achievable in a conventional manner. While transcystic cholangiography is easily performed through the gall bladder fundus (puncture site seals well), many surgeons prefer passing the needle through the liver, via the gall bladder bed into the gall bladder. However, as for biopsy, slight pressure by a blunt instrument or pledget should control most biopsy bleeds.

Problems and solutions

- Complications of laparoscopy in general.
- Difficult access in a scarred abdomen (see section on Access, pages 22, 30).
- Bleeding during access, manipulation and biopsy in liver disease.
- In ascites, floating bowels and omentum, and the volume of ascitic fluid make access and creation of the pneumoperitoneum difficult and hazardous (injury to bowel, excess pressure). Ensure that the ascites is removed before inducing a pneumoperitoneum or frothing will obscure the view, or use an open laparoscopy technique.
- In acute intestinal obstruction, there is a high risk of intestinal perforation and lack of space for pneumoperitoneum and inspection.

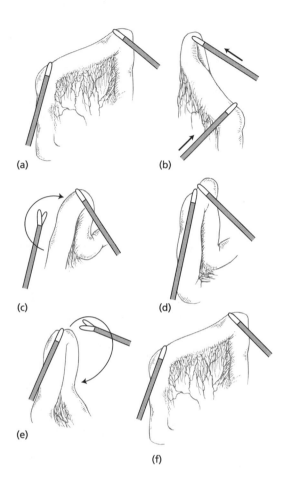

(a)

(b)

(c)

(d)

(e)

(f)

Fig. 88 Walkabout of small bowel. (a,b) Inspect both surfaces of bowel and mesentery; (c,d) release one grasper and re-grasp near the second; (e,f) release second grasper and re-grasp further along the intestine.

Here, any attempt at laparoscopy must be via an open technique.

• Bleeding from the biopsy site and bile leakage from cholangiography. Make sure the sites are dry before completion of laparoscopy.

• In severe trauma valuable time may be lost if the patient is not carefully selected.

• Minilaparoscopy through fine cannula and telescope under local anaesthetic may not be tolerated by some patients, so an experienced anaesthetist should be in attendance.

Laparoscopic ultrasonography

Contact ultrasonography is a highly sensitive and specific means of exploring the abdomen in open surgery. Its diagnostic accuracy has been found to be superior to transabdominal scanning and computerized tomography for hepatic and pancreatic malignancy.

To enhance the surgeon's ability to explore and evaluate anatomic structures, contact sonography has now been developed for laparoscopic imaging. The ultrasound probes usually employ linear curved array technology incorporated into a 10 mm probe (fits 10 mm cannula) which has a flexible tip in one or two directions. The probes are also capable of colour flow and pulsed Doppler ultrasonography.

Advantages

• To assess surgical anatomy, and detect and stage cancer of the liver, pancreas, retroperitoneum, gynaecological organs, colon and stomach.
• To assess bile duct anatomy and residual stones, thus avoiding the need for cholangiography.
• In cancer surgery, laparoscopic ultrasound may influence surgical decision making and reduce operating time. For example, if the portal vein is involved in pancreatic cancer at laparoscopic ultrasonography, resection is not feasible.

Disadvantages

• Requires a learning curve.
• Complete contact between the probe and the tissue may be limited by the number and site of the laparoscopic cannulae.
• The method is less effective than cholangiography in the investigation of the ampulla, because the dynamic study, which can be obtained by cholangiography, is not possible by ultrasonography.
• Cost.

Laparoscopic adhesiolysis

Indications

• To obtain access during any laparoscopic procedure.
• Adhesiolysis for chronic or recurrent abdominal pain.
• As an emergency to relieve obstruction.

Instruments

• Three cannulae (3.5–12 mm).
• An angled telescope (30/45°) may prove very helpful. A 0° telescope may be adequate.
• Two atraumatic, grasping forceps, preferably insulated.

- Scissors, preferably insulated with double-action curved thin blades.
- Fine hook or needle monopolar diathermy.
- Bipolar diathermy may occasionally help.
- Suction and irrigation (separate or incorporated with diathermy).
- Additional instruments for combined procedures.

Preparation

- Nasogastric intubation, and a urinary catheter may be needed.
- Where to expect adhesions:
    (a) Existing abdominal wall scar;
    (b) Site of previous surgery and inflammation;
    (c) Pre- and per-operative ultrasound studies.

Technique

In adhesioloysis, the number, size and site of cannulae is dependent on the size of the patient, extent of adhesions, and nature of other laparoscopic procedures that need to take place at the same time. Generally, the open technique of laparoscopy is preferred. The primary cannula should be placed well away from the abdominal scars. This will allow a panoramic view of the operative field, and safe access for the secondary cannulae, usually on the same side of the telescope (Fig. 89). A change of telescope from the primary to a secondary cannula may improve exposure and instrument access.

As for open surgery, determine the anatomy first, and then stretch adhesions before division. Avoid stripping if possible. Adhesiolysis is best performed with scissors through the least vascular areas. However, tough adhesions require monopolar needle/fine hook diathermy or the ultrasound activated scalpel or shears. Bleeding

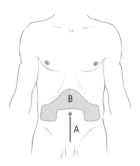

Fig. 89 Position of cannulae for adhesiolysis in the lower abdomen. A, Lower midline scar; B, site for the primary and secondary cannulae.

vessels should be coagulated with diathermy (monopolar or bipolar) or ultrasound scalpel. Suction and irrigation often are needed to clear smoke and clots.

Problems and solutions

- Complications of laparoscopy in general.
- Inappropriately positioned cannulae:
  (a) Too close to the scar to see adequately or work instruments.
  (b) Working instruments opposite the telescope or obscured by the adhesions.
  Here re-siting of the cannula or placing other cannulae may solve the problem.
- Establishing the anatomy may be difficult because of dense or complex adhesions and/or poor imaging from smoke and bleeding. In this situation consider conversion to a laparotomy.
- Bleeding from extensive adhesiolysis may disturb laparoscopic imaging. Meticulous technique and continuous suction/irrigation minimizes this problem.
- Visceral injury from handling and diathermy that might become apparent per- or postoperatively requires immediate attention.

Laparoscopic cholecystectomy

Laparoscopic cholecystectomy has, over the past 10 years, evolved to become the standard procedure for symptomatic gallstones. The majority of cholecystectomies are now performed via this route but certain preconditions must apply before this should be undertaken. These are as follows:

- There must be no evidence of biliary obstruction as determined by the liver function tests. Transabdominal ultrasound should always be performed to confirm the diagnosis of gallstones and exclude the presence of intra- and extrahepatic biliary dilation.
- The patient must have proven gallstones as the cause of their symptoms.
- There must be no evidence of portal hypertension which may make the procedure hazardous.
- There must be no contraindication to tension pneumoperitoneum.

There are two dominant areas of controversy relating to laparoscopic cholecystectomy other than those which relate to the performance of laparoscopic surgery in general. The first controversial area revolves around the need for per-operative cholangiography. The second area questions the feasibility and practicality of laparoscopic exploration of the common bile duct if common bile duct stones are found. The following narrative describes a 'middle ground' approach which represents the current majority view. It can however, be contested on a number of fronts.

Indications

The indications are no different from those for conventional open cholecystectomy.
- Gallstones causing:
  (a) Recurrent biliary colic;
  (b) Gallstone pancreatitis;
  (c) Acute cholecystitis (caution is required here—the operation may be straightforward if performed within the first 2 days of an acute attack. Beyond this time point and certainly by seven days after the onset of the attack. the operation is difficult and hazardous and if attempted, conversion rates will be high. Even at open operation there is considerable risk of bile duct injury).
- Gall bladder polyps.

Instruments

- Two 5 mm cannulae.
- Two 10 mm cannulae.
- Reducers for 10 mm cannulae.
- End-viewing 10 mm laparoscope.
- Two grasping forceps, one of which may have teeth for grasping the fundus of a chronically inflamed, thickened gall bladder wall.
- Dissecting scissors (curved).
- Hook diathermy probe.
- Toothed grasping forceps (10mm) for removal of the gall bladder via the conventional route.
- Re-usable or disposable clip applier.
- Suction/irrigation device.
- Retrieval bag if required.
- Pre-formed knotted loops (e.g. the 'endoloop') may be required if the cystic duct is too wide to accept clips.

Preparation

- General anaesthesia with muscle relaxation and epidural anaesthesia if appropriate.
- Patient in the supine position but with the patient secured to the

operating table in such a manner as to facilitate upwards and lateral tilting.
• Nasogastric intubation to decompress the stomach for the duration of the operation if necessary. This is usually removed within 6 h of the completion of the cholecystectomy.
• Urinary catheter is required only if a protracted procedure is envisaged (e.g. laparoscopic exploration of the common bile duct).

Technique

Intravenous prophylactic antibiotics are administered with the induction of anaesthesia. The operating surgeon stands on the patient's left-hand side and the assistant/camera operator on the patient's right. The pneumoperitoneum is established by open insertion of the first intraperitoneal cannula in the infra-umbilical position. Further 5 mm and 10 mm cannulae are inserted under direct vision according to the surgeons's individual practice. In general this will consist of a 10 mm cannula in the subxiphisternal position just to the left of the mid-line (Fig. 90), a subcostal 5 mm cannula about

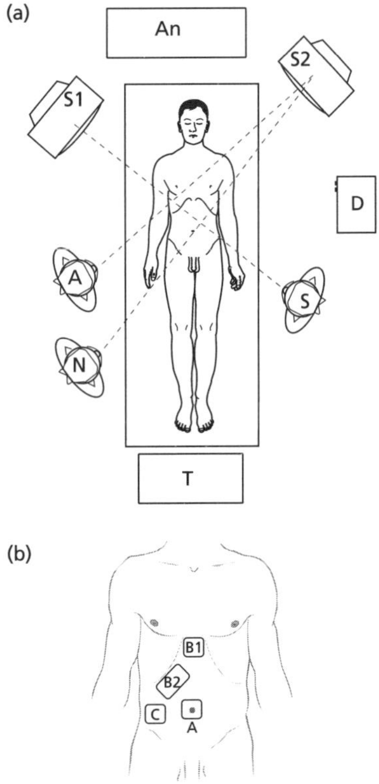

(a)

(b)

Fig. 90 (a) An example of theatre layout for cholecystectomy. (S) Surgeon; (A) assistant; (N) nurse; (S1, S1) screens (T) instrument trolley; (An) anaesthetic apparatus; (D) diathermy/US/laser.
(b) Position of cannulae. (A) Telescope; (B1, B2) working cannulae; (C) grasper to fundus or retractor.

a handsbreadth to the right of the epigastric cannula in the anterior axillary line, and a forth cannula in the right iliac fossa in the midaxillary line. The patient is placed in a head-up tilt and rotated slightly to the left. A 5 mm grasper is inserted via the right iliac fossa port and grasps the fundus of the gall bladder so that the assistant can push this cephalad to facilitate exposure of the peritoneal fold overlying the inferior border of the cystic duct. Using a 5 mm grasper through the right upper quadrant cannula to exert traction on Hartmann's pouch and diathermy scissors through a 5 mm reducer placed over the 10 mm epigastric cannula, the surgeon divides any omental adhesions to the gall bladder. Applying traction to Hartmann's pouch the peritoneal fold over the cystic duct is divided, sweeping this peritoneum in the direction of the common bile duct. Using a combination of sharp and blunt dissection the junction between the cystic duct and common bile duct is cleared. *The use of diathermy in this angle is prohibited.* Further dissection of Calot's triangle continues until the origin of the cystic duct from the gall bladder has been identified and the anatomy clearly defined, ensuring that there is no common right hepatic duct inserting directly in the cystic duct. In the course of the dissection the cystic artery will have been identified and may be safely clipped (using two clips on the proximal side and one on the gall bladder side) and divided between the clips (Fig. 91).

At this stage some surgeons routinely perform an operative cholangiogram by clipping across the proximal cystic duct, performing a cholecystodochotomy and inserting a cholangiogram catheter passed via a wide-bore needle inserted at a convenient point through the abdominal wall. After insertion of the catheter into the cystic duct it is secured there by the loose application of a further clip onto the cystic duct more proximally over the catheter. After performing the cholangiogram and confirming (or otherwise) the absence of stones in the common bile duct, this clip can be removed, the catheter taken out and the cystic duct secured with two further clips prior to its division. If a stone is found in the common bile duct, then a number of alternative options are available and are detailed below. However, it is believed by the advocates of routine per-operative cholangiography that the X-rays serve not only to determine the presence of stones in the common bile duct but, perhaps more importantly, provide reassurance that the anatomy has been correctly recognized and that no important structures have been inadvertently clipped or divided. There is little evidence to support this view and 'non-cholangiographists' would claim that the risk of failing to identify common bile duct stones in patients who have had previous pan-

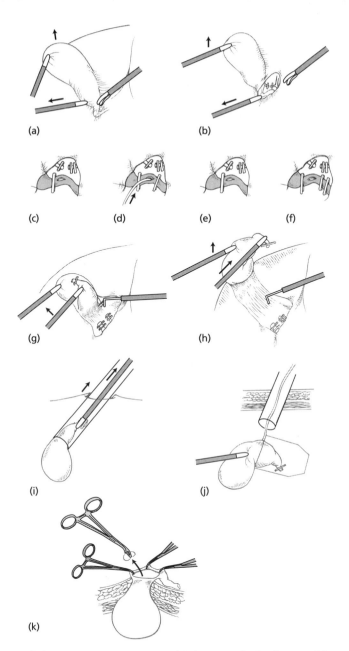

Fig. 91 Cholecystectomy. (a) Dissection of Calot's triangle; (b) clipping of the cystic artery and defining of the cystic duct; (c) clipping of the cystic duct and a small opening in the cystic duct for the cholangiogram; (d) cholangiogram catheter secured by a loose clip; (e) the loose clip and catheter removed; (f) cystic duct secured with two proximal clips before division; (g) dissection of the gall bladder from the hepatic bed; (h) haemostasis while the gall bladder is attached at fundus; (i) the gall bladder is pulled into the cannula which is then withdrawn above the skin; (j) or the gall bladder is retrieved within a bag; (k) gall bladder or retrieval bag is held at the cannula site where it is grasped, opened, emptied and removed.

creatitis or jaundice, and have normal liver function tests and ultrasonography, is vanishingly small and can in any event by safely left to be dealt with at endoscopic retrograde cholangiopancreatography (ERCP) without risk of cystic duct leaks. Moreover, biliary damage during laparoscopic cholecystectomy has usually occurred before the cholangiogram has been performed.

Once the cystic duct and cystic artery have been divided, the gall bladder can be dissected from its hepatic bed using diathermy scissors. Here, however, the diathermy hook can be used to advantage. It is a useful trick to leave the gall bladder attached to the liver at the fundus until all haemostasis has been secured in the gall bladder bed, for once the gall bladder has been completely excised from its bed, all opportunities for upwards liver traction have been lost and haemostasis can be difficult to obtain. When the gall bladder is free, a large toothed grasper is inserted via the 10 mm epigastric cannula to hold the gall bladder securely by the cystic duct in order to manoeuvre it through the epigastric 10 mm cannula site for extraction from this incision. The cystic duct and Hartmann's pouch are pulled into the cannula which is then withdrawn, leaving Hartmann's pouch protruding above the skin level at the port site where it is grasped with a haemostatic clip and opened. The liquid contents of the gall bladder are aspirated and the gall bladder retrieved by gentle traction through the port site, crushing the stones if necessary to permit removal of the gall bladder. After checking that the operative field is bloodless and dry, the cannulae are removed under direct vision to ensure that branches of the epigastric arteries have not been injured during trocar/cannula insertion. The pneumoperitoneum is released and the 10 mm cannula sites closed with a J-needle suture. It is unnecessary to insert drains.

Problems and solutions

• Excessive adhesions and inflammatory tissue obscure the anatomy. Convert to an open procedure.
• Bleeding from the cystic artery. This can often be secured laparoscopically by experienced surgeons. Avoid pointing the arterial jet at the lens. Press on the site with a convenient instrument without attempting to grasp the bleeding point. Aspirate any blood, so as to prevent light absorption. If the situation is under control, wait a few minutes, prepare a clip and on removal of the compressing instrument the artery will often have clotted and this provides sufficient time to apply a haemostatic clip. *Do not apply clips or diathermy blindly in this area*. If after one attempt to control the bleeding this procedure

fails, or if the bleeding cannot be rapidly controlled by local pressure, convert to an open procedure.

• The gall bladder is inadvertently opened during dissection from the liver. Escape of bile is of little consequence and can readily be aspirated from the peritoneal cavity at the end of the procedure. The freed gall bladder can be placed in a retrieval bag for removal without further contaminating the peritoneal cavity. The escape of stones from the gall bladder is a little more problematical. An attempt to capture all the stones should be made. Again, a retrieval bag is helpful. Soft stones may disintegrate in a grasper and these can be removed by repeated suction/lavage. There is no evidence that the occasional stone lost in the peritoneal cavity ever caused any harm.

• Bile duct injury evident at the time of laparoscopic cholecystectomy. Convert immediately. Seek the assistance of a surgeon experienced in bile duct reconstruction.

• Gall bladder too distended to permit purchase of a grasper. A needle can be inserted through the abdominal wall and into the gall bladder to aspirate the contents.

• The cystic duct is too wide to accept conventional clips prior to division. Larger diameter clips are available but it may be better under such circumstances to divide the cystic duct, place the loop of a preformed knotted loop over a grasper and then grasp the open cystic duct with this grasper prior to sliding the loop down the shaft of the grasper and around the cystic duct (Fig. 92). Take care not to tent up the common bile duct during the tightening of this knot around the cystic duct. An alternative is to complete mobilization of the gall bladder without dividing the cystic duct and then slip the knotted loop over the fundus of the gall bladder down to the cystic duct. Two further endoloops can be similarly placed to secure the proximal and distal ends of the duct before dividing the cystic duct between the ligatures after they have been tightened.

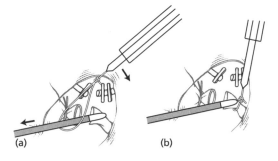

Fig. 92 Ligation of the cystic duct with a preformed knotted loop (pretied ligature).

(a) (b)

Complications

- General complications of laparoscopic surgery and biliary surgery.
- Shoulder pain occurs in about 40% of patients. Real cause unknown. Usually settles within 24 h. If persistent, perform ultrasound to exclude biliary leak.
- Development of jaundice. Indicates a major bile duct injury until proven otherwise. (The other possibility is common bile duct obstruction by a stone which has slipped into the duct.) Perform an ultrasound or CT scan to determine whether or not there is a subhepatic collection. If so drain percutaneously and proceed to direct imaging of the biliary tree via ERCP and/or percutaneous transhepatic cholangiogram to determine the extent and level of the injury. Refer to a surgeon experienced in biliary reconstruction. Strictures may be managed by stenting. If the jaundice is caused by a stone, this can be retrieved by sphincterotomy and basket or balloon retrieval at ERCP.
- Subhepatic collection without jaundice. May be due to a missed accessory duct to a clip slipping from the cystic duct. A percutaneous drain should be inserted and an ERCP performed to determine the nature of the biliary leak. Provided there is no duct obstruction, accessory ducts usually close spontaneously. If the leak is caused by a slipped cystic duct clip, this may be replaced at re-laparoscopy, or a stent may be placed at ERCP and left in until the cystic duct occludes.

Management of common bile duct stones

If a stone is discovered at cholangiography during routine laparoscopic cholecystectomy, the surgeon has three options:

1 Perform a laparoscopic exploration of the common bile duct. This is a protracted and technically complex procedure which requires the use of a 5 mm choledochoscope and double imaging system. The cystic duct is dilated and the 5 mm choledochoscope inserted to identify the stone. This can be retrieved with a balloon. An alternative procedure, similar to that used at conventional open cholecystectomy for supraduodenal exploration of the common bile duct, may be employed. Laparoscopic exploration of the common bile duct is technically demanding.

2 Convert to an open procedure and perform a conventional supraduodenal exploration of the common bile duct.

3 If the common duct is not dilated and the stone is small or questionable, it may be better to leave the stone *in situ* and perform a subsequent ERCP and sphincterotomy and remove the stone via this route.

Appendicectomy

Indications

- All stages of acute appendicitis including perforation and mass.
- Interval appendicectomy and recurrent abdominal pain.

Instruments

- Three to four cannulae (3.5–12 mm).
- Reducers for large cannulae.
- One, preferably two, end-viewing or angled telescopes (10 mm and 5 mm).
- Two or three atraumatic grasping forceps.
- One traumatic (toothed) forceps.
- One dissecting scissors (additional suture cutting scissors are an advantage).
- One hooked diathermy probe, or bipolar forceps, or ultrasound activated scalpel/shears.
- Suction and irrigation.
- One suture or endoloop introducer.
- Two or three endoloops or a piece of absorbable suture material.
- One needle holder.

Preparation

- General anaesthesia with muscle relaxation.
- Patient in supine position.
- Nasogastric tube at the anaesthetist's discretion and in peritonitis.
- Urinary catheter only if the bladder is not empty or difficult to palpate as in obese patients.

Technique

The technique of insertion of the Veress needle and/or primary cannula (closed or open method) and creation of a pneumoperitoneum are described previously. A 10 or 12 mm periumbilical primary cannula allows the appendicectomy to be carried out via a 10 mm telescope (straight or angled), and extraction of the appendix without contamination of the wound. Slow CO_2 insufflation is preferable and a pressure of 8–10 mmHg is usually adequate. First, inspect the peritoneal cavity and confirm the diagnosis, degree of appendicitis and position of appendix, before deciding where to put the secondary

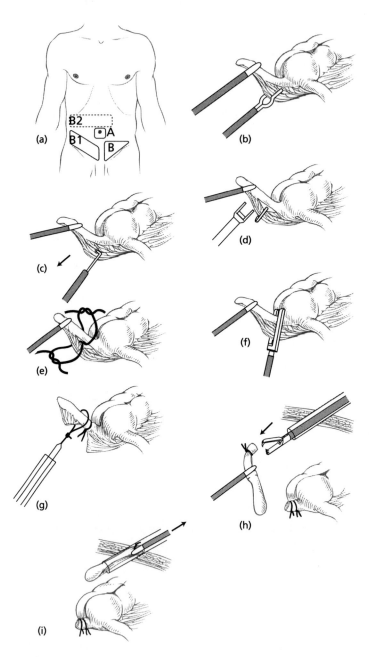

Fig. 93 Laparoscopic appendicectomy. (a) Position of cannulae. (A) primary for telescope and removal of appendix; (B and B1) two working cannulae, one of which may also be used for removal of appendix; (B2 a fourth cannula for retraction if necessary. (b,c and d) Securing mesoappendix with bipolar diathermy, unipolar hook, clip or high energy ultrasound. (e,f) Securing both mesoappendix and appendix by suture ligatures or linear stapler-cutter. (g) Securing appendix by pretied loops. (h,i) Appendix removed through a cannula—usually 10 mm or more.

working cannulae. For most appendicectomies, two 5 mm lower abdominal secondary cannulae are all that are required (Fig. 93). However, in difficult cases or with an awkward retrocaecal/ileal appendicitis a third right, but high, secondary cannula allows retraction of bowel (caecum). In order to facilitate exposure, the patient is then placed in the Trendelenburg position with left lateral tilt. However, tilting may allow spread of infective matter particularly in localized lower abdominal peritonitis or the presence of an appendicular abscess. The appendix is gradually mobilized using a combination of blunt and sharp dissection until its tip can be clearly identified and grasped. Sometimes, the dissection and/or the appendicectomy has to be performed in a retrograde manner. The mesoappendix is identified and divided using bipolar diathermy and scissors, or hook monopolar diathermy, or one or two suture ligatures (Fig. 93). The recently developed, ultrasound-activated scalpel/shears may prove more effective. Three absorbable suture ligatures or endoloops are placed around the base of the appendix and secured prior to division of the appendix, leaving two sutures on the appendix stump. Alternatively, bipolar coagulation at the site of the division obliterates the lumen and a single suture to the base secures the appendix stump. Other approaches to secure both the mesoappendix and appendix include using a linear stapler–cutter or endoclips (Fig. 93).

Hold the free appendix near its transected end by an atraumatic grasper in the left hand. Remove the 10 mm telescope, but place a 5 mm telescope through the other secondary cannula (the one nearest to the surgeon). A 5 mm reducer is now placed into the peri-umbilical cannula and a 5 mm toothed forceps is then passed to grasp the transected end of the appendix. The free appendix is removed through the 10–12 mm primary cannula without contamination by infected material. The 10 mm telescope is replaced and the abdominal cavity carefully inspected for safe completion of the procedure. Any identified pus is suctioned out under vision and, if preferred, the operating field or the entire peritoneal cavity lavaged with warm saline and antiseptic solution. A purse-string or a Z suture is necessary when the ligation of the base is thought to be difficult or inadequate as in cases of perforation or gangrene near the base. The cannulae are removed as described earlier (page 60) and the pneumoperitoneum is evacuated completely prior to the last cannula removal. Fascial incisions greater than 5 mm are closed carefully (using the purse-string/anchoring suture on a J-needle as described for an open laparoscopy). The patient's hospital stay is determined by the nature of the appendicitis in the first place. Patients undergoing an interval appendicectomy may be discharged from the hospital after 24 h.

Problems and solutions

- Awkwardly positioned or difficult appendectomy:
  - (a) Use a third secondary cannula;
  - (b) Try an angled telescope (30 or 45°);
  - (c) Convert to an open technique.
- In pelvic or high appendicitis, very low and/or close to each other secondary cannulae may be difficult to use because of restriction to instrument movement and an inappropriate distance between the cannulae and the target area (too close for pelvis and too far for right upper quadrant). Here, change of cannula site or an additional cannula in a more appropriate site may help.
- Partially obstructed and distended loops of bowel which are stuck to the site can be difficult to manipulate and the bowel may be damaged.
  - (a) Tilt the table.
  - (b) Use blunt instruments (rounded end atraumatic grasper or sucker probe), as fingers in open surgery, to sweep rather than pull the bowel away from the inflammatory mass.
- Spread of pus.
  - (a) Un-tilt the operating table.
  - (b) Suck away all infective materials immediately.
  - (c) Carefully lavage the peritoneum before completion.
- Tense or friable appendix may fall apart and contaminate.
  - (a) Careful handling;
  - (b) Suction immediately.
- Bipolar coagulation will not obliterate the lumen of a severely inflamed, friable or tense gangrenous appendix.
- Determining the anatomy may be difficult because of imaging problems or the advanced nature of the appendix mass. Here, convert to an open technique.
- Bleeding from mesoappendix:
  - (a) Careful and adequate coagulation;
  - (b) Suction/irrigation may be required;
  - (c) In difficult appendicectomies, apply a suture ligature or an endoloop.
- Cannula, instrument and diathermy injury to viscera (small bowel, caecum, right iliac vessels, ureter, gonadal vessels, right tubo-ovary).
- Appendix too big or friable to come out easily through the 10 or 12 mm cannula. Here, use a retrieval bag with or without wound extension (see page 92).
- The patient may experience postoperative pain from three sources:
  - (a) Cannula site (short duration, avoid local infiltration of

anaesthetic agent in peritonitis);

(b) Pneumoperitoneum (avoid rapid insufflation, and high pressure if possible and evacuate gas completely after completion);

(c) Peritoneal irritation from the inflammatory process which takes a few days to settle.

- Wound infection:

   (a) Avoid contamination;

   (b) Antiseptic/antibiotics may help.

- Stump leakage. A potentially serious complication which can occur immediately or in up to several days after surgery caused by:

   (a) Loose ligature. Double ligature or an additional Z suture/purse-string minimizes this risk.

   (b) Coagulation near the base devitalizes tissue. Avoid both bipolar and monopolar diathermy for 1 cm from the base at all times and avoid monopolar diathermy after ligation of the base (Fig. 94).

   (c) Severely diseased or perforated base. Apply a purse-string or a Z suture.

   (d) Very tight suture ligature or clips may cut through the tissue particularly with a very diseased or tense appendix.

- In difficult cases a drain tube may minimize the effects of stump leakage.

Complications

Complications are the general complications of laparoscopy and conventional surgery including inadequate appendicectomy, intra-peritoneal septic collections and incisional hernias.

Laparoscopic Nissen's fundoplication

Indications

- Failed antireflux medical treatment.
- Potential long-term use of proton pump inhibitors.

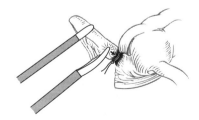

Fig. 94 Monopolar scissor diathermy cut after ligation of the appendix allows energy concentration and burn at the base.

- Patients with complications of gastro-oesophageal reflux.
- Adjunct to repair of complex (types II or III) hiatus hernias.
- Adjunct to insertion of gastrostomy in paediatric patients with vomiting.

Contraindications

- In reflux associated with significant oesophageal shortening.
- In patients with reflux caused by oesophageal dysmotility conditions such as scleroderma.
- Carcinoma of the oesophagus.

Instruments

- Five cannulae (3.5–12 mm) with appropriate reducers.
- One 30–45° telescope (additional zero degree telescope may be an advantage).
- Liver retractor.
- One soft Babcock or soft bowel clamp to grasp the stomach or oesophagus.
- Two atraumatic, preferably insulated, curved grasping forceps (one may be right-angled).
- One curved insulated dissecting scissors (additional suture cutting scissors are an advantage).
- Unipolar diathermy (additional bipolar diathermy or ultrasound scalpel/shears are an advantage).
- One toothed grasping forceps with ratchet for holding the sling.
- One piece of nylon tape or plastic tube.
- One needle holder (a second needle holder for suturing is an advantage).
- Appropriate non-absorbable suture materials on needles (ski, straight or curved needles).
- Suction and irrigation.
- Clips and clip applicator (particularly when short gastrics are to be divided).
- Retractor arm to hold the liver retractor if assistants are unavailable.

Preparation

- General anaesthesia with muscle relaxant.
- Wide-bore NGT.
- Patient in supine position with a degree of head-up tilt.

- Surgeon stands between the legs (the hip joints preferably non-flexed) with the camera operator on the patient's right side (Fig. 95). If lower limb abduction is not possible, the surgeon may stand on either side of the patient.

Technique

The cannulae site and sizes are modified according to individual anatomy and size. In general (Fig. 95), a 10–12 mm primary cannula is inserted at, or a few centimetres above, the umbilicus for the telescope. A 5–10 mm cannula is placed on the right adjacent to xiphoid sternum for the liver retractor. One 5 mm cannula in the right upper quadrant and one, preferably 10 mm cannula, in the left mid or upper quadrant (10 mm cannula allows a medium sized ordinary curved needle through for suturing). A 5–10 mm cannula in the left mid/lower abdomen is used for traction of the stomach and a sling. This cannula may also be used for holding the wrap in place during suturing.

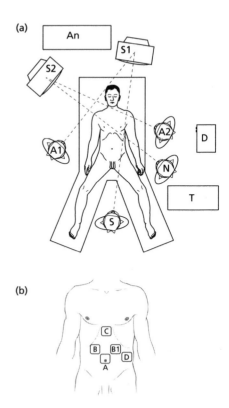

Fig. 95 Laparoscopic Nissen fundoplication. (a) Theatre layout. (S) Surgeon; (A1 and A2) two assistants; (N) nurse; (S1, S2) two screens; (T) instrument trolley; (An) anaesthetic apparatus; (D) diathermy or ultrasound and suction/irrigation. (b) Position of cannulae. (A) primary for telescope; (B, B1) two working cannulae; (C) retractor; (D) grasper for traction on stomach and sling.

Mobilization of the oesophagus, repair of the hiatus and fundoplication are performed in an identical fashion to that of a conventionally performed operation (Fig. 96). A window is made in the gastrohepatic omentum and continued upwards towards the hiatus. This occasionally involves clipping and dividing the hepatic branch of the anterior vagus nerve. Care must be taken to divide any accessory left hepatic artery (arising from the left gastric artery) between clips as this may bleed profusely if not clipped. Division of the gastro-hepatic omentum reveals the right crus of the diaphragm from which the oesophagus (or lesser curve of the stomach if a sliding hiatus hernia is present) should be dissected. The left crus is mobilized as per the open operation and, using an angled telescope, the window between posterior stomach/oesophagus and the left crus is identified and opened, care being taken to preserve the posterior vagus nerve intact. A sling may then be passed round the oesophagus and used to retract the oesophagus/stomach to complete the dissection. Ligation of the short gastric vessels is usually unnecessary, however, this may be accomplished either by doubly clipping individual vessels and dividing between clips or, if available, by use of the high energy ultrasound device (shear). The gastric fundus is then manoeuvred behind the oesophagus and a 240° (Toupet) or 360° (Nissen) fundo-plication performed by suturing the fundus to the oesophagus or itself as appropriate (after the first stitch, the sling may be removed). A #40 bougie in adults is passed to ensure that the wrap is not too tight. A posterior crural plication is usually necessary to prevent migration of the wrap into the mediastinum. If required, as in paediatric patients, a gastrostomy may be fashioned via the laparoscope or a combined laparoscope and endoscope. At the end of the procedure, the pneumoperitoneum is evacuated completely and all fascial defects greater than 5 mm are sutured. Postoperative intravenous or epidural analgesia may be required for the first 12 h, however, local infiltration of the wounds with appropriate anaesthetic agents at the end of the procedure may provide adequate pain relief.

Fig. 96 (*Opposite*) Laparoscopic fundoplication (arrows indicate direction of traction and instrument movement). (a) Dissection through the gastrohepatic omentum which continues towards and around the hiatus. (b) Dissection of the oesophagus from the right crus. (c) The left crus is revealed. (d) A window is created behind the oesophagus. (e) A curved/angled grasper placed behind the oesophagus. (f) A sling is passed around the oesophagus. (g) Completion of the dissection behind the oesophagus. (h) Hiatus repair. (i,j) The gastric fundus is manoeuvred behind the oesophagus. (k, l) Suturing of the fundus. (m) A complete tension free 'floppy' wrap.

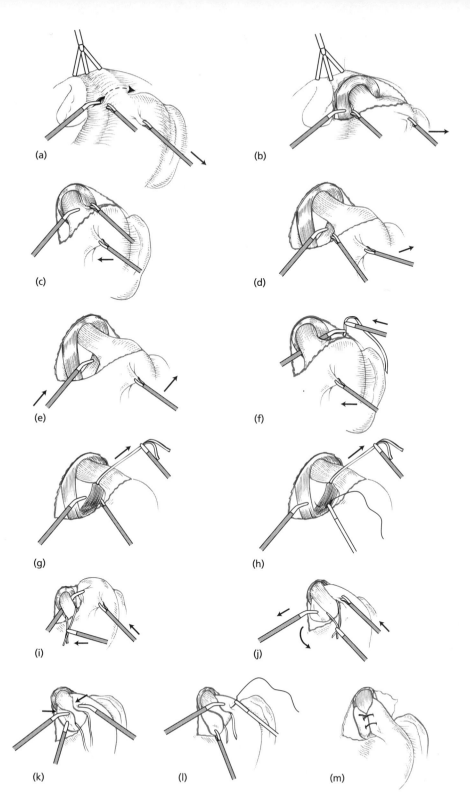

The patient may be fed at 24–48 h postoperative and discharged home on day 3 or 4.

Problems and solutions

- General complications of laparoscopy and surgery.
- In obese patients the procedure can be very difficult. Pre-operative weight reduction is highly recommended.
- Large hiatus hernia and significant peri-oesophagitis increase the risk of oesophageal injury, minor bleeds and injury to vagi nerves. Techniques are available to close the hiatus with patches of synthetic material.
- Short oesophagus prevents adequate mobilization of the oesophagus and fundoplication. It also increases the risk of recurrent hiatus hernia.
- Distended transverse colon, large liver or large spleen can make access and safe instrumentation hazardous.
- Liver injury from retraction and the suturing needle are not uncommon. Therefore extreme care and appropriate retraction are essential.
- Gastro-oesophageal injury during traction and mobilization can happen particularly when the surgeon is inexperienced.
    (a) Avoid grasping the oesophagus, but if required, use either a soft or large Babcock.
    (b) Manipulate the oesophagus by pushing with the side of an instrument in the required direction, gentle traction of the stomach or traction on a sling.
    (c) Use a soft bowel clamp or a soft Babcock to manipulate or retract the stomach.
- Pneumothorax. During mobilization of the posterior aspect of oesophagus, there is a tendency to dissect deep to the opposite crus. The risk of pneumothorax is increased in the presence of hiatus hernia or short oesophagus.
- Extracorporeal knotting can lead to tissue damage by serration and knot sliding. Therefore, internal knotting is preferred.
- The risk of knot sliding may be further reduced by using braided suture materials.
- Complications as for conventional open Nissen's fundoplication.

Laparoscopic gastroenterostomy

There have been a number of modifications and innovations in the instrumentation available for advanced laparoscopic procedures which have enabled the performance of several procedures which would otherwise not have been feasible. Thus the development of laparoscopic linear stapler–cutters, laparoscopic bowel clamps, expandable fan retractors and instruments capable of curving within the peritoneal cavity to enable retraction of circular organs such as the oesophagus or colon have all stimulated surgeons to attempt increasingly more complex procedures such as antireflux surgery, gastroenterostomy and laparoscopic colorectal surgery. All of these advanced laparoscopic procedures are predicated on the ability to perform intracorporal laparoscopic suturing which remains the 'quantum leap' of manual dexterity which is required before advanced laparoscopic procedures can be pursued (see page 78). Laparoscopic gastroenterostomy is one of these procedures which requires familiarity with the technique of laparoscopic suturing.

Indications

- Gastric outflow obstruction caused by carcinoma of the pancreas.
- Gastric outflow obstruction caused by unresectable carcinoma of the gastric antrum confirmed radiologically, ultrasonically and laparoscopically.
- Gastric outflow obstruction caused by pyloric stenosis resulting from chronic duodenal ulceration (associated with laparoscopic truncal vagotomy) in a patient who is unsuitable for a conventional open operation. However, it is important to appreciate that under such circumstances the procedure would contravene conventional wisdom insofar as the gastroenterostomy is placed in the anterior wall of the stomach as opposed to a posterior gastroenterostomy which would be the normal accompaniment of a truncal vagotomy. However, there are few clinical trial data to support the perceived wisdom.

Preparation

- Ensure full correction of the metabolic alkalosis associated with pyloric outflow obstruction and the fluid imbalance which may accompany pyloric stenosis. These metabolic changes may influence the tolerance of the myocardium to the tension pneumoperitoneum.
- Perform gastric lavage for as long as is feasible pre-operatively in order the ensure that the stomach is as clean and empty as possible at the time of the procedure.
- Plan the procedure carefully. The positioning of the access ports for this operation (see below) is critical and the presence of adhesions

from previous abdominal surgery through vertical abdominal incisions may mean that it is not possible to perform this procedure. Facility with open laparoscopy as previously described is mandatory for this procedure because of the required positioning of the ports.

• The patient must be firmly secured to the operating table in the modified Lloyd-Davies position. This is important because extreme positive and negative Trendelenberg angles may be required to identify the duodeno-jejunal flexure and then facilitate the apposition of the afferent loop to the greater curve of the stomach. The hip joints must be non-flexed (or even minimally extended) to enable the operating surgeon to stand between the patient's abducted thighs without the surgeon's movements being frustrated by the patient's thighs, as for a laparoscopic Nissen's fundoplication (Fig. 97).

• The procedure may be somewhat protracted and so the insertion of a bladder catheter is a prudent precaution. Moreover, the insertion of the primary port is such as to necessitate a completely empty bladder so as to avoid puncture of this organ.

(a)

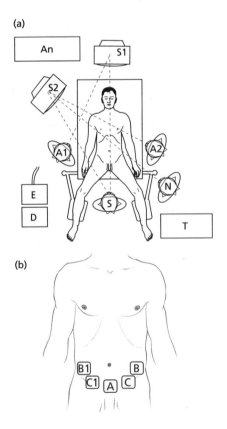

(b)

Fig. 97 Laparoscopic gastroenterostomy. (a) Patient position. (S) Surgeon; (A1 and A2) two assistants; (N) nurse; (S1 and S2) two screens; (T) instrument trolley; (D) diathermy; (E) suction/irrigation; (An) anaesthetic apparatus. (b) Position of cannulae. (A) Primary for telescope; (B and B1) for graspers; (C) for grasper and first needle holder; (C1) for second needle holder and stapler).

Instruments

- Four 10 mm diameter cannulae.
- One 12 mm diameter cannula to receive the linear stapler–cutter.
- Appropriate 5 mm reducers.
- Two or three atraumatic graspers (add rubber-shod for holding sutures).
- Two 5 mm diameter needle-holders for suturing.
- A 30° telescope in addition to the conventional end-viewing telescope.
- One 5 mm pair of scissors.
- Fine diathermy hook or needle.
- A 5 mm suction/irrigation probe.
- 3/o diameter Vicryl sutures.
- 35 mm linear stapler–cutter loaded with an intestinal (as opposed to vascular) cassette. Two further cassettes will be required.
- Number 0 or 1 Vicryl on a J-shaped needle for closure of the port sites.

Technique

After preparation on the skin and appropriate draping of the patient, open insertion of the first cannula is conducted in the midline suprapubically. It is important to appreciate that the positioning of the cannula sites (Fig. 97) for this procedure is deliberately low down in the abdominal wall, because in the conditions for which this procedure is conducted the stomach is frequently distended and enlarged to below the level of the umbilicus. Thus, the conventional site of insertion of the cannula used for the insertion of the telescope would make it impossible to visualize the stomach and infracolic compartment. Having completed a full laparoscopic examination of the peritoneal cavity, accompanied wherever possible by laparoscopic ultrasonography to confirm the nature of condition being treated, the remaining cannulae are inserted. These consist of a 10 mm cannula in the left iliac fossa and two further 10 mm cannulae in each flank at the level of the umbilicus. A 12 mm cannulae is inserted into the right iliac fossa and corresponding 5 mm reducers are applied to each cannula. The iliac fossa cannulae are for the insertion of the needle holders (5 mm diameter) but the 12 mm cannula in the right iliac fossa is specifically for the insertion of the linear stapler–cutter at the appropriate moment.

The first manoeuvre is to determine whether or not there is

sufficient anterior gastric wall (in patients with gastric cancer) to perform the procedure laparoscopically. A useful tip is to use a 5 mm diameter grasper marked at 5, 10 and 15 cm intervals to compare with the available free or non-infiltrated gastric antrum. A gastroenterostomy needs to be at least 7–10 cm long and so for the present purposes there must be least 15–20 cm of free greater curve to work with. Having established that an appropriate free length of greater curve and anterior gastric wall are available for the anastomosis, the operating table is tilted strongly into a head-down position, and two 5 mm graspers inserted through the right and left iliac fossa cannulae. The transverse colon is manipulated in a cephalad direction and the duodenojejunal flexure identified. The jejunum is then traced aborally until a point which is 30–40 cm beyond the duodenojejunal junction has been reached and this is then manipulated to the greater curvature of the stomach (Fig. 98). The patient is then tilted into an extreme head-up position whilst holding the appropriate point of the jejunum in one of the graspers. This allows the stomach to fall towards the pelvis and brings it within range of needle holders inserted through the iliac fossa cannulae. A further grasper is then inserted through the left upper cannula to replace the grasper holding the jejunum and thus free up the two cannulae in the iliac fossae for the insertion of needle holders. Thus, the grasped point on the jejunum is sutured to the greater curvature of the stomach and a further stay suture is used to approximate the stomach and jejunum at a further point 10–12 cm distal to the first stay suture. These stay sutures are cut about 2–3 cm long so that they can be held by graspers inserted through the two upper cannulae. This enables the application of counter-traction during insertion of the linear stapler–cutter.

With the two stay sutures placed on tract, an anterior gastrostomy and jejunostomy are performed close to the distal stay suture. A 35 mm linear stapler–cutter is then inserted through the 12 mm cannula in the right iliac fossa and passed upwards and to the patient's left, one jaw of the instrument being inserted into each of the enterotomies. The stapler–cutter is closed and fired and then withdrawn and re-loaded. The procedure is repeated to produce a gastroenterostomy of 6–7 cm in length. An alternative is to use a single firing of a 60 mm linear stapler. When this stage of the procedure has been completed this leaves a diamond-shaped defect at the site of the gastrostomy and jejunostomy, which is closed with a continuous suture, each stitch being held under tension by an assistant using a grasper inserted through the left upper port.

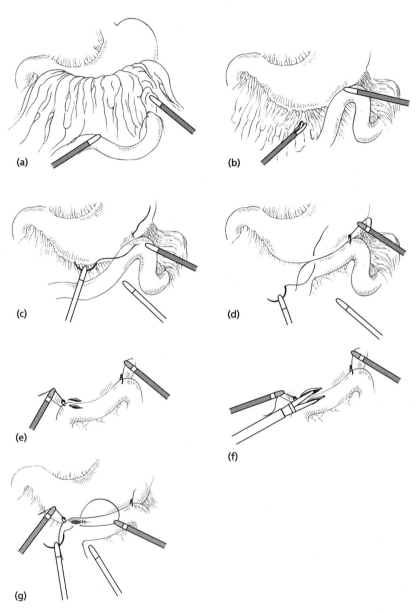

Fig. 98 Laparoscopic gastroenterostomy. (a) Patient in head-down position when an appropriate site for the anastomosis identified; (b) in extreme head-up position the proximal end of the anastomosis site on the stomach and jejunum are approximated; (c) a stay suture at proximal point; (d) the second stay suture at the distal point; (e) an anterior gastrostomy and jejunostomy close to the distal stay suture to accommodate the stapler; (f) the stapler in place; (g) the defect at the site of gastrostomy and jejunostomy is closed. Use graspers with rubber-shod jaws to keep tension on all suture materials.

Problems and solutions

• Difficulties with making the gastrotomy and jejunotomy. Using diathermy scissors or fine probe, the seromuscular layer is incised so that the mucosa protrudes. This can then be 'tented' up using a curved atraumatic type of gasper and an oval of mucosa removed using curved diathermy scissors. Bleeding is rarely troublesome with this technique and there is very little in the way of spillage from the enterotomies.

• Difficulties inserting the jaws of the linear stapler into the gastrotomy and jejunotomy. In addition to applying counter traction to the stay sutures, an atraumatic grasper can be used to hold the orifices of the enterotomies open so as to facilitate insertion of the jaws of the stapler.

Complications

• General complications of laparoscopy and conventional surgery.
• Bleeding from the stapler line.
• Bleeding and leakage from the suture line — hence the importance of keeping this suture under tension at all times during the suturing.

Truncal vagotomy and highly selective vagotomy

These procedures for chronic peptic ulcer are rarely undertaken, given the efficacy of modern medical therapy. Those who are adept at laparoscopic Nissen's fundoplication (see page 125) will have no difficulty in mobilizing the gastro-oesophageal junction and hiatal area to identify the anterior and posterior vagal trunks. The anterior vagus can readily be isolated from the anterior wall of the oesophagus with a diathermy hook and then divided using this same instrument. However, the posterior vagus nerve frequently contains a substantial blood vessel and it is more prudent to divide the nerve between clips. After truncal vagotomy a drainage procedure is mandatory and the simplest one to perform is the anterior gastro-jejunostomy described above (see page 130). It should be borne in mind that an anterior gastrojejunostomy defies conventional wisdom insofar as at open surgery it is conventional for this to be a posterior gastrojejunostomy.

The necessity for a gastric drainage procedure can be avoided by using one of the modifications of the highly selective procedure which appears not to disrupt the pyloro-antral emptying mechanism. The anterior nerve of Latarget is traced from its origin from the anterior vagus and all the branches which it sends to the lesser curvature of the stomach are divided down as far as the leash of blood vessels of the gastric incisura known as the 'crow's foot', keeping the main trunk on the nerve of Latarget intact. These branches run with the blood vessels supplying the lesser curvature of the stomach which must therefore be individually dissected free and divided between clips in such a manner as to denude the anterior portion of the lesser curve as far as the lower 4 cm of the oesophagus, ensuring the integrity of the anterior vagus nerve and the nerve of Latarget. This process can be tedious and time consuming and a technique has been described whereby a linear stapler can be used to perform this part of the procedure, working from the 'crow's foot' up the lesser curve seriatim, but again, care must be taken to avoid damage to the main nerve of Latarget. If the vagotomy is to be completed as conventional highly selective vagotomy, the surgeon continues to work his way around the lesser curve of the stomach to divide those nerves (and blood vessels) in the middle and posterior leaves of the gastrohepatic omentum close to the stomach in order to avoid damage to the main trunk of the posterior nerve of Latarget.

An alternative and much less time consuming procedure to the conventional highly selective vagotomies is to perform a posterior truncal vagotomy and anterior leaf highly selective vagotomy. This appears to possess all the attributes of the conventional anterior, middle and posterior left highly selective vagotomy but is less tedious to perform. Some authors have modified this even further by suggesting that the anterior highly selective vagotomy may be substituted by an anterior gastric seromyotomy and claim equally effective results.

Laparoscopy for perforated duodenal ulcer

Indications

The indications are as for conventional open surgical intervention for perforated anterior ulcer.

Instruments

- Four cannulae (5, 10 and 12 mm) with appropriate reducers.
- One end-viewing or preferably a 30° telescope.
- One liver retractor. (Suction/irrigation probe or an atraumatic grasper may provide adequate retraction).

- Two atraumatic graspers.
- One dissecting scissors (insulated).
- Unipolar diathermy (an additional bipolar diathermy is an advantage).
- One needle holder (additional second needle holder is an advantage).
- Absorbable suture ligatures and sutures on a needle (3/o Vicryl).
- Suction and irrigation.

Preparation

- General anaesthesia with muscle relaxant.
- NG tube.
- Patient in supine position.
- Surgeon stands either between the legs or one side of the patient.

Technique

Figure 99 illustrates the position of the cannulae. The technique for insertion of the Veress needle and the primary cannula (peri-umbilical) are dependent on the surgeon's preference, and the presence of peritoneal adhesions and the presence of significant ileus. In general, it is safer to use an open technique for laparoscopy. Confirm the diagnosis via the telescope before insertion of the secondary cannulae. If necessary, place one of the lateral secondary cannulae first and use a suction and irrigation to aspirate the peritoneal fluid, and gently lift the liver edge and sweep the fibrinous adhesions to establish the nature of the perforation and its suitability for laparoscopic suturing or omental patch, or both. At this stage, a degree of head-uptilt may improve exposure. Half-circle round-bodied or tapered needles on 3/o Vicryl or Dexon can be used through a 10mm cannula for interrupted intracorporeal suturing technique (stronger material may be used on either slightly straightened-out needle or a ski needle). Repair of the perforation, with or without an omental patch, and

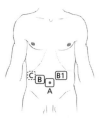

Fig. 99 Position of cannulae for perforated duodenal ulcer. (A) Primary cannula for the telescope; (B and B1) two working cannulae for suturing; (C) a fourth cannula may be used for retraction of liver or colon, suction/irrigation, or holding omental patch.

peritoneal toilet are performed in a fashion similar to that of a conventionally performed operation (Fig. 100). At the end of the procedure, if required, a small drain may be inserted through the right cannula site.

Definitive laparoscopic surgical treatment of a benign peptic ulcer, involving some form of vagotomy is dependent on the surgeon's preference and expertise, the patient's condition and the duration of perforation as with conventional open surgery.

Postoperative care and the need for opiate analgesia are dependent on the patient's general condition and the degree of peritonitis prior to surgery.

Problems and solutions

• General complications of perforated duodenal ulcer, laparoscopy and surgery.
• Difficult access caused by advanced peritonitis, adhesions and distended bowel.
    (a) Open laparoscopy technique may reduce the risk of insertion of Veress needle/primary cannula.
    (b) A fourth cannula (third secondary cannula) may allow adequate bowel retraction (transverse colon).
• Adequate peritoneal toilet can be a problem because of occlusion of the suction probe by omentum, appendices epiploicae, loops of bowel, and large particles of food debris. Use large sump suction with patience.

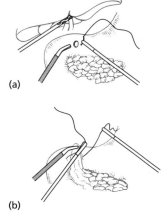

Fig. 100 Suturing of perforated ulcer, (a) without or (b) with omental patch. Note the suction probe is used as a liver retractor.

(a)

(b)

Laparoscopic splenectomy

Indications

A difficult procedure, most suitable for small-sized spleens as in idiopathic thrombocytopenic purpura and Hodgkin's disease (as part of the staging procedure which includes liver and lymph node biopsies).

Instruments

- Five cannulae (5, 10, and 12mm).
- Appropriate number of reducers to 5mm (some cannulae have built-in reducers).
- One 0° and one angled (30 or 45°) telescopes.
- One curved double jaw action scissors (additional hooked scissors are an advantage).
- Two atraumatic, preferably insulated, curved grasping forceps and a third with a ratchet.
- Both bipolar and unipolar hook diathermy. Alternatively ultrasound activated shears.
- One retractor.
- One soft Babcock or bowel clamp to grasp stomach, colon, omentum and splenic pedicle.
- One 10mm reusable, or preferably 5 or 10mm multifire automatic disposable clip applicator.
- Suture ligature.
- Suction and irrigation device.
- Retrieval bag.

Preparation

- General anaesthesia with muscle relaxation.
- Supine position with a moderate head-up and a degree of lateral tilt (the patient needs to be well supported and strapped to the table if a steep lateral tilt position is preferred).
- A nasogastric tube is necessary.
- The surgeon and one assistant should stand on the right-hand side of the patient (Fig. 101).

Technique

The primary (telescope) cannula is placed a few centimetres above and to the left of the umbilicus (Fig. 101). The site and size of the secondary working cannulae may be modified slightly depending on the size and shape of the patient (obese, small and thin, angle of the costal margin), and the preference of the individual surgeon. A Babcock or bowel clamp is placed through the lower right cannula to grasp and retract the body of the stomach downwards and to the right. This puts the greater omentum on stretch, thereby exposing the spleen.

First, divide the splenocolic attachments around the lower pole of the spleen to the back of the organ until the lower margin of the lienorenal ligament is reached using a combination of bipolar or low monopolar coagulation diathermy or ultrasound shears, scissors, sutures and clips as required (Fig. 102). Then divide the gastrosplenic (short gastric vessels) attachment using clips and/or suture ligature or ultrasound shears. At this stage, some surgeons advocate clipping or ligating the main splenic artery in continuity just above the pancreas, a few centimetres away from the spleen. This will interrupt

(a)

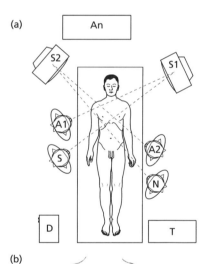

(b)

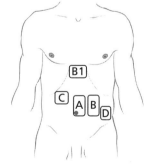

Fig. 101 Splenectomy. (a) Theatre layout; (S) surgeon; (A1, A2) assistants; (N) nurse; (S1, S2) screens; (T) instrument trolley; (D) diathermy or alternative energy source; (An) anaesthetic apparatus. (b) Position of cannulae; (A) primary cannula for telescope; (B, B1) working instruments; (C, D) working instruments or retractor. The telescope may be moved from one cannula to another to improve viewing.

most of the blood supply to the spleen, thereby reducing the risk of major haemorrhage and diminishing the size of the spleen through spontaneous venous drainage. This may or may not follow ligation

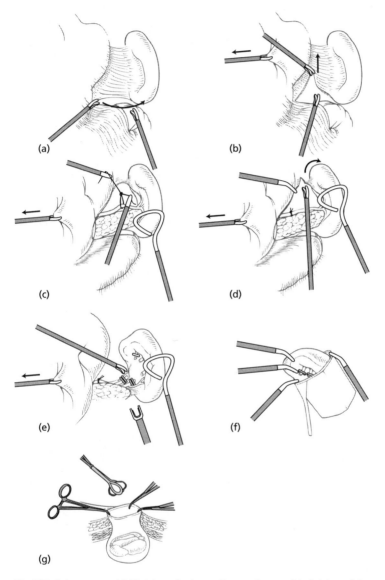

Fig. 102 Splenectomy. (a) Division of splenocolic attachment; (b) division of short gastric vessels; (c) ligation of the splenic artery without vein in continuity; (d) mobilization of the superior attachments; (e) dissection and division of the hilum followed by the retroperitoneal attachments; (f) removal of the spleen in a strong impermeable bag; (g) fragmentation and extraction of the spleen in a partially exteriorized bag.

of the main splenic vein. Division of the gastro-oesophagophrenic peritoneal reflection and mobilization of the upper pole of the spleen is effected by scissors and diathermy. At different stages of the procedures, the spleen may have to be retracted in different directions using a liver fan retractor or an endoflex retractor through either the epigastric cannula or the most lateral cannula on the left. Dissection now proceeds towards the hilum of the spleen. The tail of the pancreas is identified and extreme care must be taken to avoid inadvertent injury to the pancreas and splenic capsule, and traction avulsion injury to the hilar vessels. All blood vessels should be clearly identified and clipped or ligated thrice (two proximal and one distal).

The retroperitoneal attachments of the spleen are then divided by scissors and diathermy or ultrasound scalpel. Before extraction, a thorough inspection is made to ensure haemostasis and to exclude accessory spleens. A strong plastic bag (retrieval bag) is placed into the peritoneal cavity via one of the larger cannulae. The isolated spleen is then placed inside the bag and the neck is exteriorized through a slightly extended cannula site. The spleen may then be fragmented by a grasper or scissors before extraction. However, if the splenectomy is performed as a staging procedure (Hodgkin's disease) an intact spleen has to be delivered through an appropriately enlarged port site or a strategically placed small abdominal incision. The cannulae are removed, the pneumoperitoneum is evacuated, and cannula sites greater than 5 mm in diameter are closed in the usual fashion. The patient may be fed within 24 h postoperatively, and discharged home at 72 h.

Problems and solutions

- General complications of laparoscopy and open surgery.
- Appropriate positioning of patient and cannulae are absolutely critical.
- Retraction of the spleen during the latter stages of the procedure can be difficult and frustrating.
- Large spleens can be very difficult to manipulate. However, the procedure can be made easier and probably safer by a preliminary identification and ligation of the splenic artery above the pancreatic border.
- Bleeding from traction avulsion of small veins or splenic tear are common.
- Placing the detached 'large' spleen into a retrieval bag can be a daunting task, and extraction of an intact average spleen requires a 3–5 cm long incision.

Laparoscopic colorectal surgery

Laparoscopic surgery for diseases of the colon and rectum has been one of the more controversial applications of the innovations which have resulted from the technological revolution surrounding laparoscopic surgery. The controversy ranges from the relatively mild, e.g. resectional versus non-resectional rectopexy for rectal prolapse, versus the extremes of dogma, e.g. the completeness of surgical resection of colorectal cancer. The purpose of this section is not to resolve the controversies which are the subject of clinical trials, but to briefly describe some of the techniques being studied. It should be emphasized that at the time of writing, in the opinion of the authors, these techniques should not be applied outside the context of a clinical trial. Accordingly we would not necessarily advocate them as the procedure of choice.

Indications

These are no different from those for conventional open colorectal surgery but the most common indications for performing these procedures are as follows:
- Inflammatory bowel disease:
  (a) Crohn's disease of the ileocaecal region;
  (b) Long-standing ulcerative colitis;
  (c) Sigmoid diverticular disease.
- Colorectal cancer. Unquestionably the single most controversial application of laparoscopic technology (see below). With the possible exception of cancer of the middle third of the rectum and of the transverse colon, all tumours of the colorectum are amenable to laparoscopic mobilization and laparoscopically assisted resection. The controversy surrounds not the feasibility but the desirability and oncological safety.
- Rectal prolapse.
- Laparoscopically assisted stoma formation (ileostomy, loop or end-colostomy in the left iliac fossa).

Contraindications

The presence of large bowel obstruction is a contraindication.

Instruments

- Cannulae of 10–12mm are used throughout. Wherever an

intracorporeal circular stapled anastomosis in the rectosigmoid region is to be performed a 30 mm cannula is required in order to be able to insert the anvil of the circular stapling device which is passed transanally. In general the average colorectal dissection will demand four to five cannulae of which one may need to be of 12 mm diameter to facilitate insertion of the linear stapler divider.

- Appropriately sized reducers for these cannulae.
- End-viewing and 30° angle 10 mm laparoscope.
- 5 mm diameter grasping forceps, of which at least two and possibly three will be required.
- Babcock's forceps — disposable or reusable. These are invariably of 10 mm diameter although 5 mm versions are available.
- Dissecting scissors (curved).
- Hooked monopolar diathermy probe (additional bipolar diathermy and ultrasound shears are an advantage).
- Reusable or disposable clip applier.
- Disposable or reusable linear stapler–cutter 35 mm in length which can accept both vascular and intestinal cassettes, the former being required for major arterial structures and the mesentery.
- Laparoscopic intestinal clamps are available and may be required wherever an intracorporeal anastomosis is being contemplated.
- Suction/irrigation device.
- Retrieval bag if a totally laparoscopic resection is being considered.
- Needle holders and sutures when a totally laparoscopic resection is contemplated (usually for benign disease).

Preparation

There should be no difference between the preparation of a patient for laparoscopic procedure and that of a conventional open operation. All patients require the usual bowel preparation, prophylactic antibiotics and pre-operative stoma siting when necessary.

General anaesthesia is required for the pneumoperitoneum. The combination of balanced anaesthesia, epidural anaesthetic, forced early enteral nutrition and very early mobilization has enabled some workers to routinely discharge patients undergoing laparoscopic colorectal resection within 2 days of operation, even in high risk patients over the age of 70 years.

The patient should be placed supine in the modified Lloyd-Davies position in all instances with the possible exception of a planned right hemicolectomy which may usually be performed without the Lloyd-Davies position. The Lloyd-Davies position is essential from several perspectives.

1   It enables an assistant to be placed between the patient's legs for the purposes of retraction and instrument holding.
2   It permits intra-operative colonoscopy to be performed simultaneously with laparoscopy to localize those lesions which are not evident on the serosal surface of the bowel, thus ensuring that the correct segment of bowel has been mobilized.
3   For those patients requiring a rectocolic anastomosis, the Lloyd-Davies position is required for trans-anal insertion of a circular stapling device.

As with all advanced laparoscopic procedures the patient must be securely strapped to the operating table to enable extreme levels of vertical and lateral tilting to be achieved in order to cause the small bowel to gravitate away from the operative field to avoid damage to it and facilitate visualization of the bowel being mobilized.

Nasogastric intubation is usually required for only a matter of a few hours for a successfully completed laparoscopically assisted procedure.

Most laparoscopic or laparoscopically assisted colorectal operations tend to be protracted procedures and thus bladder catheterization is a useful precaution. It can usually be removed within 24 h of the operation.

Technique

Clearly, the technique to be employed will be determined by the nature and extent of the procedure to be undertaken and details of individual procedures are beyond the scope of this text. However, for operations on the right colon, a supra- or infra-umbilical cannula will provide adequate visualization of the peritoneal cavity to enable the insertion of 10 mm cannulae into the left upper quadrant, right upper quadrant and left lower quadrant. Appropriately inserted graspers or Babcock forceps then allow sufficient traction to be exerted on the tissues to enable dissection of the right colon over to the midline, the surgeon, camera-holding assistant and theatre nurse all standing on the patient's left with the video monitors being placed on the patient's right. Once the right colon has been sufficiently mobilized over to the origin of the right colic artery, ileocolic artery and right branch of the middle colic artery, the decision may be made to divide these intracorporeally with a linear stapler divider; or to simply make a small transverse incision in the right upper quadrant of the abdominal wall, through which the surgical specimen is prolapsed, and the vascular pedicles divided extracoporeally and divided and ligated in the usual fashion. The bowel can then be divided in the conventional manner and an anastomosis performed in the preferred fashion extracorporeally.

Intracorporeal anastomosis can be performed after laparoscopic-assisted right hemicolectomy, using the triangulation technique. This is tedious and time-consuming and it is doubtful that it significantly diminishes overall hospital stay.

For left hemicolectomy the side from which the team work is reversed and on this occasion a 12 mm cannula is inserted in the suprapubic position. This enables the insertion of the linear stapler–cutter if necessary. For patients undergoing rectal excision for rectal cancer, the laparoscopic visualization of the mesorectum for the purpose of total mesorectal excision is exceptionally good but does require familiarity with the open technique of total mesorectal excision before it can be satisfactorily practised via the laparoscope. Here, the 30° angled telescope can really come into its own for identification and preservation of the pelvic nerves, particularly in the narrow male pelvis. It should be emphasized that this dissection is not for the occasional rectal (or laparoscopic!) surgeon.

During the dissection of the rectosigmoid, division of the congenital adhesions between the colon and parietal abdominal wall is achieved readily through the laparoscope and permits identification of the left ureter in the intersigmoid fossa. The plane of dissection of the descending colon is achieved by incising superiorly in this plane until the left phrenocolic ligament is reached. This can frequently be obscured by the small bowel and requires extreme tilting of the patient vertically and to the right, causing the small bowel to gravitate into the pelvis. This same is true for mobilization of the hepatic flexure except that the table is tilted to the patient's left. It is the segment of bowel between the two flexures which poses the greatest problem for the laparoscopic surgeon, for division of the gastrocolic omentum is difficult and tedious. Whilst it is certainly possible to mobilize the transverse mesocolon close to the bowel in patients with inflammatory bowel disease, to do so in a patient with transverse colon cancer risks compromising the lymphatic oncological margins of resection and, with present technology, is deemed unwise.

For diseases of the sigmoid, descending colon and rectum, full mobilization of the splenic flexure is readily achieved laparoscopically, as is division of the appropriate vessels, particularly the inferior mesenteric artery, using the vascular cassette of a linear stapler–cutter. Similarly, the right colic and ileocolic arteries can be similarly divided intracorporeally. Having achieved this the bowel can also be transected, but most surgeons who undertake this form of surgery prefer to stop at this point, perform an appropriately sited transverse incision, and prolapse the whole of the mobilized colon/rectum on the surface of the abdominal wall and complete the resection and anastomosis extracorporeally.

For patients with rectal prolapse the options lie between resectional rectosigmoidectomy and laparoscopic mesh rectopexy. The details of these procedures may be found in specialized texts, but there is some rationale in mimicking laparoscopically the operation which appears to provide optimal results when performed as an open operation, i.e. resection rather than rectopexy. However, the disadvantage of this may be a greater complication rate, particularly with regard to the incidence of ureteric injury, the reasons for which are obscure.

Problems and solutions

- Injury to the bowel during the traction required for dissection. 5 mm graspers are preferable to avoid this complication. However, *under no circumstances should the bowel in the region of a tumour, or the tumour itself be directly grasped with an instrument.* It is preferable to grasp the adjacent fat and mesentery to avoid this complication. The use of an assistant to apply counter-traction to the tissues is essential in this type of laparoscopic surgery.
- Injury to vital structures: the ureter, duodenum or iliac vessels. Convert to an open procedure immediately if this is suspected.
- Difficulty identifying structures because of the presence of adhesions. This may occur even in the absence of previous surgery. It is a matter of persisting carefully with adhesiotomy or, because of time constraints, converting to an open approach if necessary.
- Difficulty in dissection because of tumour adherence to another organ—convert immediately.
- Difficulty in identifying structures because of obesity. The presence of excess fat in the mesentery may prevent adequate dissection— convert to an open operation.
- The bowel may be over-distended by the bowel preparation, thus making it difficult to perform the dissection for fear of perforating the bowel. On-table colonoscopy to decompress the bowel may help.
- Failure to identify a mucosal lesion on the peritoneal surface of the bowel. Simultaneously laparoscope and colonoscope the patient to identify the site of the lesion to ensure that the correct segment of bowel is mobilized and removed. The diseased site (carcinomatous polyp, etc.) may be marked by the injection of methylene blue at the base of the lesion in such a way that the dye becomes visible on the serosal surface at laparoscopy. Alternatively this may be performed

24 h before operation in order to avoid per-operative distension of the colon, which can be troublesome to decompress at the time of the operation.

Complications

- Complications of laparoscopic surgery and colorectal surgery.
- Port site herniae—indicate the universal necessity to routinely close all port sites of 10 mm diameter or more with a J-needle, particularly the subumbilical port site.
- Port site recurrences of colorectal cancer. The significance of this complication has yet to be proven in a controlled clinical trial. Opinions vary between no added risk and a threefold risk of wound recurrence.
- There is no consensus as to the relative risks of laparoscopic versus open colorectal surgery. Fears of an increased risk of deep venous thrombosis and pulmonary embolus from a protracted operating time have not been supported by meta-analyses—if anything the reverse is true. However, the potential advantages need to be confirmed or refuted by randomized clinical trials.

Laparoscopy for undescended testes

Indications

Impalpable testes (unilateral). The management of bilateral impalpable testes should be undertaken by specialists in the field.

Instruments

- Up to three cannulae (3.5–5 mm) with appropriate reducers. A 10 mm cannula may only be required if 10 mm telescope or 10 mm clip applicators are used.
- One 3.5 or 5 mm, 0 or 30° telescope.
- One dissecting scissors, preferably insulated.
- Two atraumatic graspers (3.5 or 5 mm)
- One atraumatic grasper with ratchet.
- Unipolar diathermy.
- 2/0 non-absorbable suture ligature (alternatively 5 or 10 mm clip applicator and clips).

Preparation

Always consent for laparoscopic and open ligation of testicular vessels, orchidopexy or orchidectomy.
- General anaesthesia with muscle relaxant.
- Patient in supine position.
- Urinary catheter only if there is a palpable bladder.
- Skin preparation to include scrotum.

Technique

The majority of patients are managed in the first few years of life, hence the open method of laparoscopy is preferred. However, in older children, particularly those who are over 10 years of age, blind insertion of the Veress needle and a primary peri-umbilical cannula are considered safe. A pneumoperitoneum is created using 0.2 l/min CO_2 with a pressure of 6–8 mmHg. The abdominal cavity (iliac fossa and lateral wall of pelvis proper) is then carefully inspected looking for a testis or vas and vessels (Fig. 103). To facilitate exposure, Trendelenburg and lateral tilt may be required. If there are no testes

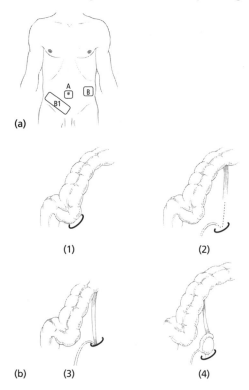

(a)

(1)

(2)

(b)

(3)

(4)

Fig. 103 Laparoscopy for undescended testes. (a) Position of cannulae. (A) primary cannula for the telescope; (B and B1) working cannulae for retraction, dissection and ligation. (b) Laparoscopic view. (1) Colon obscuring anatomy at and above the internal ring, (2) vas and vessels ending blindly above the internal ring; (3) vas and vessels entering the ring; (4) testis seen in the abdomen.

and vas and vessels are seen clearly either ending blindly or entering the internal ring, no further laparoscopic procedure is required. In the latter case, however, exploration of the groin may be undertaken to retrieve atrophic tissues ('nubbins') for histology. If the anatomy is not clear because of overlying or adherent colon, first tilt the operating table head up and laterally and then insert one or two secondary cannulae to retract or mobilize the colon.

If a testis is located, two secondary cannulae will be needed for one of the following laparoscopic procedures (Fig. 104):
• Ligation of the testicular vessels (stage one Fowler–Stephens operation). The second stage procedure (orchidopexy) can be done laparoscopically 6–12 months later.
• One-stage orchidopexy.
• Single-stage Fowler–Stephens orchidopexy (ligation of testicular vessels and orchidopexy at the same time).
• Orchidectomy:
    (a) Unilateral undescended abnormal looking testes;
    (b) Unilateral undescended testes after the age of 10 years;
    (c) Bilateral undescended testes after puberty.

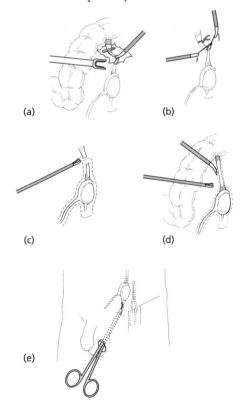

(a)   (b)

(c)   (d)

(e)

Fig. 104 Different types of procedures that can be carried out on intra-abdominal testis. (a,b) Ligation of the testicular vessels using clips or suture ligatures; (c) mobilization of testis and vas in second stage Fowler–Stephens procedure; (d) complete mobilization of testis, vas and vessels in single stage orchidopexy; (e) trans-scrotal delivery of testis medial to the inferior epigastric vessels.

Ligation of the testicular vessels is easily performed with either two non-absorbable suture ligatures, or two metal clips. For orchidectomy, the testis is mobilized, vas and vessels are ligated and divided, and the testis is removed via a cannula. Suspected malignant testes should be extracted within a strong retrieval bag.

In orchidopexy the vas is mobilized first as higher dissection may result in blood obscuring the lower operative view. The dissection may then be continued around the vessels and finally the testis itself. Leave the gubernacular attachment intact at the internal ring, otherwise the testis may fall into the pelvis or disappear between loops of bowel. At this point a dartos pouch is created and a long, thin grasping forceps (laparoscopic or conventional forceps) is passed through the scrotum, into the external ring, through the abdominal wall and into the peritoneal cavity medial to the epigastric vessels. Grasp the gubernaculum, then divide it distally before pulling the testis and its attachment through the created tunnel into the dartos pouch. Care must be taken not to injury the iliac vessels which are very close. Alternatively, a small incision above the pubic bone should allow a conventional orchidopexy. Once the conventional testicular alignment has been checked, the pneumoperitoneum is evacuated and the cannulae removed in the usual fashion. In small children, fascial defects greater than 4 mm are closed. The procedure may be performed as a day case.

Problems and solutions

- General complications of laparoscopy and surgery, and surgery for undescended testis.
- Injury to testicular vessels, epididymis and vas may occur from direct grasping. Therefore, apply the forceps to the edge of the covering peritoneum rather than the structure itself.
- There is potential for damage to the iliac vessels or ureter.
- Short vessels. In this situation, the options are:
  (a) Orchidopexy to a high point in the scrotum. A second operation to bring the testis further down, or an orchidectomy, may be required at a later date.
  (b) Divide the vessels for a two-stage or one stage Fowler–Stephens procedure (two-stage is not valid if the vas is already mobilized).
  (c) Orchidectomy.
  (d) Microvascular transfer if expertise available.
- Short vas. Transfer the testis via the most medial point, or consider orchidectomy in unilateral cases.

Varicocele

Unilateral or bilateral primary varicocele (including recurrent varicoceles).

Instruments

- Three cannulae (3.5–10 mm) with appropriate reducers.
- 3.5 or 5 mm end-viewing telescope.
- Two curved atraumatic grasping forceps (one needs to be fairly pointed with insulation).
- One dissecting curved scissors.
- One 5 or 10 mm clip applicator and clips (alternatively non-absorbable suture ligature materials).
- Bipolar or monopolar diathermy

Preparation

- General anaesthesia with muscle relaxants.
- Patient in supine position.
- Urinary catheter only if the bladder is palpable.

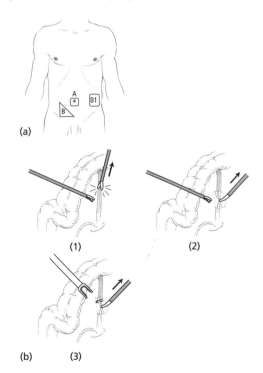

Fig. 105 Ligation of left varicocele. (a) Position of cannulae. (A) primary for telescope; (B and B1) two working cannulae. (b) Ligation with clips. (1) Identify the vessels well above the internal ring and lift up the overlying peritoneum before making a small incision using scissors; (2) using two fine, preferably angled, atraumatic forceps to gently isolate the testicular —two or more veins; (3) one or two clips/ligature complete the procedure.

Technique

Figure 105 illustrates the sites of the cannulae and procedure. A pneumoperitoneum is created using CO_2 at a low flow rate and a pressure of 8–10 mmHg. The testicular vessels are identified well above the internal ring. A degree of head-down and lateral tilt improves exposure. Occasionally, minor adhesions between colon and iliac fossa require division. The peritoneum over the vessels is incised for 1 cm, and the veins (usually two with a few other small venules) mobilized sufficiently to allow the application of one or two metal clips or non-absorbable suture ligatures. Abnormally large vas-associated veins are carefully isolated and ligated. In recurrent varicoceles, and when difficulties are experienced in separating the veins from the artery, both veins and artery may be ligated.

The operative area (iliac fossa) is then inspected to ensure all collateral veins have been identified and controlled with diathermy (preferably bipolar). The pneumoperitoneum is evacuated and the cannulae are removed in the usual fashion. The patient may be treated as a day case.

Problems and solutions

- Complications of laparoscopy and surgery in general.
- Often difficult to identify the testicular artery.
- Bleeding from traction avulsion of testicular veins.
- Management of abnormally dilated vas associated veins must be by minimal and careful dissection.
- Potential for injury to iliac vessels and ureter.
- Scrotal emphysema can occur rarely, but resolves spontaneously.
- Persistent/residual varicocele because of incompletely ligated veins or collaterals.
- The risk of testicular dysfunction after ligation of both veins and artery in humans is uncertain.

Laparoscopic simple nephrectomy

Indications

- Small dysplastic/scarred non-functioning kidney.
- Multicystic dysplastic kidney.
- Non-functioning hydronephrotic kidney.

The role of laparoscopic simple or radical nephrectomy in the management of neoplastic kidneys is highly controversial.

Instruments

- Four or five cannulae (3.5–12 mm) and appropriate converters.
- One end-viewing telescope (an additional 30 or 45° angled telescope is an advantage).
- One retractor.
- Two atraumatic, preferably insulated, relatively fine curved grasping forceps (an additional forceps with ratchet is an advantage).
- One traumatic (preferably with ratchet) grasping forceps.
- One curved insulated double action jaw scissors with appropriate diathermy leads.
- A diathermy (preferably bipolar) or an ultrasonic scalpel/shears.
- Suction/irrigation.
- One automatic 5 or 10 mm clip applicator and clips (a single load reusable clip applicator is usually adequate). Alternatively use suture ligatures.
- One long needle to decompress the dilated or cystic kidney if necessary.
- One retrieval bag particularly if infection, stones, or malignancy are suspected.
- A few pretied suture ligatures (endoloops) may be useful.
- Vascular endoscopic linear stapler–cutter device and tissue morcellator may be useful at the surgeon's discretion.
- One or two balloons (balloon dissector) to create a retroperitoneal space, but only for retroperitoneal nephrectomy.

Preparation

- General anaesthesia with full muscle relaxation.
- The patient is placed in the full lateral (nephrectomy position) for adults and semilateral position for children (Fig. 106).
- Bladder catheterization is performed only if the bladder is palpable, or the urine output requires monitoring.

Technique for transperitoneal nephrectomy

Figure 106b illustrates the position of the cannulae. A pneumoperitoneum is created through a Veress needle or an open technique primary cannulation. It is usually decided to insert two of the secondary working cannulae first, assess the situation and feasibility of the procedure, and then determine what size and where exactly the remaining one or two secondary cannulae should be. It is also possible that the procedure may be converted to an open procedure at this stage.

The upper part of the lateral aspect of the colon on the relevant

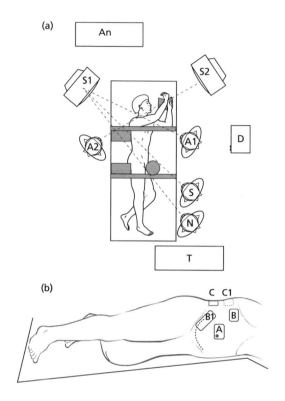

Fig. 106 Laparoscopic right nephrectomy. (a) Theatre layout. Note how the patient is fully supported and strapped. (S) surgeon; (A1, A2) assistants; (N) nurse; (S1, S2) screens; (T) instrument trolley; (D) diathermy or alternative energy source; (An) anaesthetic apparatus. (b) Position of patient and cannulae. (A) Primary for telescope and instruments; (B) secondary working cannula; (B1) secondary cannula for instrument and telescope placed laterally in the lower abdominal skin crease which may be enlarged to retrieve the specimen or carry out combined bladder surgery; (C) secondary cannula for instruments and retractor; (C1) an accessory cannula for retractor if necessary.

side is dissected from the lateral abdominal wall (Fig. 107). This allows the colon to fall medially under gravity. In paediatric patients, however, the dissection of colon may be minimal. In difficult cases, the ureter is identified first and used as a retractor, however, in multicystic dysplastic kidney and most cases of small dysplastic, refluxing and hydronephrotic kidneys, identification of the ureter in the early stages of the procedure is unnecessary.

The anterior surface, lower pole, upper pole and the medial border (hilum) of the kidney are freed in a sequential manner. To prevent the kidney from gravitating medially, leave parts of the lateral and posterior surface attachments intact until the pedicle is secured and divided. The kidney may be grasped and manipulated by either its capsule or the body (in benign fibrotic/cystic kidneys), or the pelvis in different directions using either an atraumatic grasper or a soft Babcock forceps. Care must be taken not to damage the kidney before its blood supply is secured. The upper edge of the peritoneum may be employed as a useful retractor (Fig. 107c). Small vessels may be coagulated and cut while the large renal vessels may be individually ligated using either sutures or clips (with or without addition endoloops), or secured by vascular staples (using a linear stapler).

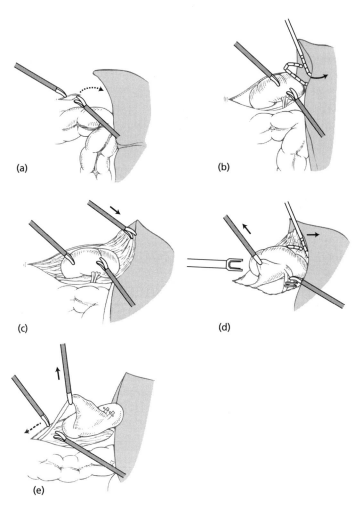

Fig. 107 Simple right nephrectomy. (a) High paracolic peritoneal incision; (b) colon falls medially, liver retracted cephalad and the kidney is exposed; (c) the upper edge of the peritoneum may be employed as a retractor; (d) superior perinephric tissues and liver are retracted cephalad while the kidney or pelvis is pulled outward to expose the renal pedicle and clipping/ligation of the vessels carried out; (e) the ureter is traced and ligated.

Once the kidney has been dissected free, the ureter is then traced, ligated/clipped and cut at an appropriate level. A dilated or cystic kidney may be decompressed at any stage of the operation. Depending on the size and nature of the pathology, the kidney may then be manipulated and extracted via a large cannula, the site of the cannula, or a retrieval bag. An appropriate size, strong and non-permeable bag allows fragmentation, morcellation or liquidization of the kidney prior to its extraction without spillage into the peritoneal cavity.

If combined surgery to the lower end of the ureter or the bladder is indicated, as in refluxing ureters, the kidney may then be left on its ureteric attachment and placed low in the retroperitoneal space created during dissection around the ureter. The specimen can then be retrieved extraperitoneally through the lower abdominal incision that is made for the second, but open part of the procedure (Fig. 108).

Patients who undergo a straightforward nephrectomy may be discharged from hospital on the first postoperative day.

Problems and solutions

- General complication of laparoscopy, surgery and nephrectomy.
- Traversing the peritoneal cavity and its related morbidity.
- Potential for injury to liver, colon, duodenum, and vena cava during a right-sided procedure, and spleen, colon and pancreas on the left.
- A chronically inflamed and adherent kidney can be difficult to manipulate, thus increasing the risk of injury to the vascular pedicle and surrounding structures.
- The role of laparoscopy in the management of a malignant condition of the kidney is questionable.
- The vesico-ureteric junction may be approached laparoscopically. However, this part of the procedure requires:
    (a) Change of patient's position;
    (b) Placement of additional cannulae;
    (c) Extensive retroperitoneal or intraperitoneal dissection.

Technique for retroperitoneal nephrectomy

The patient is placed in the renal position (as for the transperitoneal approach). A 1–2 cm incision just below the tip of the 12th rib is deepened by blunt dissection to expose Gerota's fascia, which is picked up with forceps and incised. Finger/blunt dissection is then performed to create a space around the kidney and the procedure is continued as described previously (see Extraperitoneal laparoscopy page 56) and above.

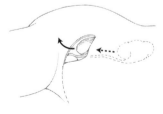

Fig. 108 Extraperitoneal approach to the distal ureter and extraction of the entire specimen (kidney and ureter) through an extended iliac fossa cannula site. This wound may be extended further if a combined bladder procedure is required.

Problems and solutions of retroperitoneal approach

See page 56.

Inguinal hernia repair

Laparoscopic approaches to inguinal hernia repair have been developed over the past 5 years but are currently undergoing assessment by clinical trial. It is as yet uncertain whether or not there are any health-care economic benefits to laparoscopic hernia repair.

The procedure may be performed transperitoneally or extraperitoneally depending on the surgeon's preference and expertise. It is absolutely crucial for the surgeon to memorize the anatomy (Fig. 109). Although femoral hernias can be repaired in a similar fashion this section describes inguinal hernia repair.

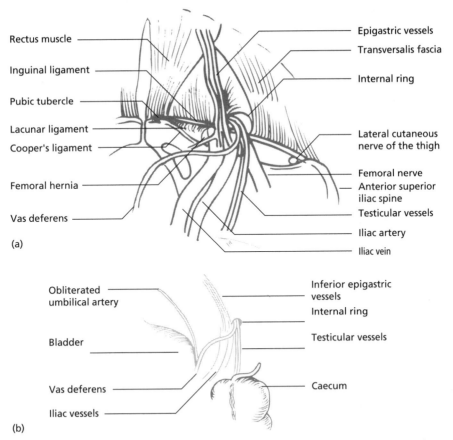

Fig. 109 Right inguinofemoral region. (a) Normal anatomy. (b) Applied normal anatomy as viewed through the laparoscope.

Indications

Unilateral, bilateral, and recurrent indirect and direct inguinal hernia.

Contraindications

General contraindications of anaesthesia, surgery and laparoscopy.

Instruments

- Three 5–12 mm cannulae with appropriate built-in or separate 5 and 10 mm converters.
- One 5 or 10 mm end-viewing, or preferably 30° angled, telescope.
- One 5 mm insulated, curved, double-jaw action, dissecting scissors with appropriate diathermy attachments.
- Two 5 mm insulated, atraumatic, preferably curved, double-jaw action, grasping forceps.
- Suction and irrigation device.
- Hernia stapler with appropriate staples (this device requires a 12 mm cannula). Alternatively, one needle holder with appropriate needle/suture materials.
- Prosthetic mesh (12 × 13 cm for unilateral repair).

Preparation

- Shaving is not necessary for this procedure.
- General anaesthesia with full muscle relaxation.
- The patient is placed in a supine position.
- Urinary catheterization is necessary if the bladder is full and in prolonged procedures.

Transperitoneal technique

The position of patient and cannulae are demonstrated in Fig. 110. The surgeon usually stands on the side opposite the hernia. However, with experience a right-handed surgeon may stand on the left side of the patient and the left-handed surgeon on the right side of the patient. A pneumoperitoneum is created using a Veress needle or preferably an open technique of primary cannulation. The patient is placed in the Trendelenburg position which allows the bowel to fall cephalad under gravity. It is essential for the surgeon to identify key anatomical landmarks (Fig. 109) which include internal inguinal ring, obliterated umbilical artery (median umbilical ligament), pubic tubercle, inguinal

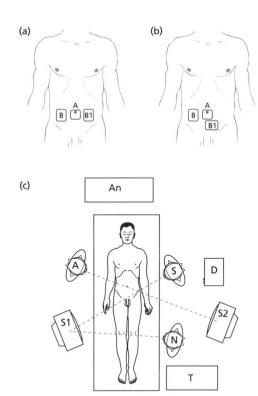

Fig. 110 Laparoscopic inguinal hernia repair. (a) Cannulae placement for hernia repair—left, right or bilateral transperitoneal, and bilateral extraperitoneal. (A) primary; (B and B1) secondary cannulae. (b) Cannulae placement for hernia repair—unilateral transperitoneal and extraperitoneal hernia (right side). (c) Theatre layout for laparoscopic hernia repair—right or bilateral hernia. (S) Surgeon; (A) assistant; (N) nurse; (S1, S2) screens; (T) instrument trolley; (D) diathermy apparatus; (An) anaesthetic apparatus.

ligament, anterior superior iliac spine, epigastric vessels, spermatic vessels, vas deferens and iliac vessels. This exercise may be facilitated by applying finger pressure externally (surgeon or assistant) on the abdominal wall over the inguinal canal while the surgeon continues to observe the screen and feels the appropriate structures with the tip of one or two atraumatic grasping forceps. The opposite inguinal region is also inspected to identify any unsuspected hernia.

A transverse incision is made in the peritoneum well above the hernial defect starting medial to the anterior superior iliac spine (lateral to the internal inguinal ring) and finishing lateral to the obliterated umbilical artery (Fig. 111). Occasionally, the obliterated ligament may have to be transected to improve access. Care must be taken not to damage the inferior epigastric vessels. This incision may be extended circumferentially at either end to incise the neck of the sac of enlarged hernias leaving the distal sac in place and thus avoiding unnecessary dissection around the cord. Care should be taken to avoid injuring the cord structures and the genital branch of the genitofemoral nerve. Using scissors and/or atraumatic grasping forceps, a lower (posterior) peritoneal flap is raised sufficiently to expose the hernial defect, inguinal ligament and Cooper's ligament (Fig. 111b). Extreme care must be taken not to injure the inferior epigastric vessels, lateral cutaneous nerve of the thigh, spermatic vessels and vas, genitofemoral nerve, iliac vessels and femoral nerve. A small hernial sac should be left intact and inverted into the peritoneal cavity. A lipoma of the cord may be excised using diathermy. Some surgeons advocate creating a window behind the spermatic cord at the level of the internal ring to fit part of the mesh. After exposing the entire inguinofemoral region, the mesh (12×13 cm for unilateral, at least twice as much for bilateral) is placed into the abdominal cavity through a 10–12 mm cannula. The mesh is then placed across the entire inguinofemoral region allowing it to drape over iliac vessels and stapled or sutured to the pubic tubercle, medial end of Cooper's ligament, rectus muscle and transversalis fascia if desired. To avoid damage to the iliac vessels, femoral nerve, cord structures and lateral cutaneous nerve of the thigh, staples or sutures are not placed below the inguinal ligament except the medial part of the Cooper's ligament that lies medial to the iliac vein where one or two staples/sutures are applied (Fig. 111c). However, there is

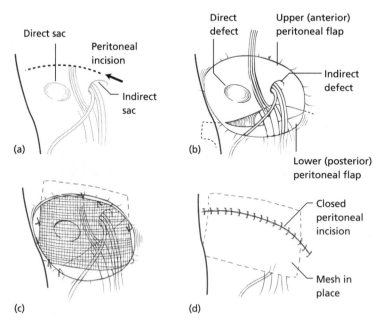

Fig. 111 Repair of right inguinal hernia. (a) Transverse peritoneal incision starts lateral to the internal ring and extends to the obliterated umbilical artery. (b) Exposure of the inguinofemoral region. (c) Mesh covering the inguinofemoral region. (d) Closure of peritoneum over the mesh.

an increasing body of evidence that supports the view that fixation of the mesh by means of staples/sutures is not necessary to achieve a successful repair. Once the mesh is in place, the edges of the peritoneal flaps are approximated and stapled or sutured over the mesh (see page 90). The pneumoperitoneum is then evacuated and the cannulae sites greater than 5 mm are closed in the usual fashion.

Extraperitoneal (preperitoneal) technique

A free preperitoneal mesh without staples or sutures is becoming an increasingly popular technique for inguinal hernia repair. The extraperitoneal space created by CO_2 at a pressure of 8–10 mmHg (range 5–15 mmHg) enables the surgeon to perform hernia repair laparoscopically and thereby avoid the morbidity that may be associated with traversing the abdominal cavity. If required, this technique can provide access to both left and right inguinofemoral regions at the same time. The approach is not suitable for those who have had previous surgery in the same extraperitoneal region. The technique of creating a pneumoextraperitoneum is detailed on page 56. In brief, a 1–2 cm skin incision is made just below the umbilicus and blunt dissection is carried out to the rectus sheath. The linea alba or the anterior rectus sheath (side of the hernia) lateral to the midline is then incised longitudinally to expose the peritoneum or the posterior rectus sheath, respectively. Care must be taken not to open the peritoneal layer. A dissecting balloon may be inserted to create the working space on the required side. Several versions are available and incorporate a channel down which the telescope may be passed in order to create the space under direct vision. Once the working space has been created, the procedure of hernia repair is continued as described above for the transperitoneal approach.

Problems and solutions

- General complications of surgery, laparoscopy and hernia repair.
- Complications of pneumoextraperitoneum (see page 56).
- Dissection or stapling injury to nerves and vessels. Care should be taken during dissection and to avoid staples or sutures at and below the inguinal ligament or altogether.

  (a) Injury to ileofemoral vessels. This can be very serious and requires an immediate open approach to repair the injured vessel.

  (b) Injury to epigastric or spermatic vessels. These may be treated by intracorporeal clipping or ligation of the vessel proximal and distal to the site of injury. Epigastric vessels may also be ligated percutaneously (see page 53–4).

(c) Injury to vas. This can be repaired by fine suturing either intracorporeally or through an open incision.

(d) Injury to the lateral cutaneous nerve of the thigh which results in transient or prolonged symptoms of numbness, paraesthesia or pain.

(e) Injury to the femoral nerve. This complication is usually transient but can be prolonged and associated with muscle weakness and atrophy in the thigh.

(f) Dissection within the inguinal canal may cause injury to the genital branch of the genitofemoral nerve, and oedema and haematoma in the inguinal region and scrotum. This complication may be avoiding by leaving the sac of large hernia in place. An extraperitoneal haematoma may be mistaken for a recurrent hernia and may be identified by ultrasound and aspirated.

- Extreme medial dissection (medial to obliterated umbilical artery) or failure to recognize the bladder especially in sliding hernia, may lead to bladder injury. The injured bladder may be repaired laparoscopically and a urinary catheter is left *in situ* for several days.

- Scrotal emphysema may occur, especially if the dissection within the canal is carried out to mobilize the distal part of a large hernia. It is a transient problem and resolves spontaneously.

- Intestinal adhesions to prosthetic mesh which is placed on the peritoneal surface (out of date technique) or where the extraperitoneal mesh has not become re-peritonealized.

- Difficultly with stapling or suturing at pubic tubercle and Cooper's ligament. Avoid using more than gentle application of the stapler or leave the mesh without any form of fixation.

- In complicated situations convert to open repair of hernia.

Index